COMPLEMENTARY THERAPIES
FOR OLDER PEOPLE IN CARE

by the same author

The Carer's Cosmetic Handbook
Simple Health and Beauty Tips for Older Persons
ISBN 978 1 84819 178 5
eISBN 978 1 84642 914 9

of related interest

Comforting Touch in Dementia and End of Life Care
Take My Hand
Barbara Goldschmidt and Niamh van Meines
Illustrated by James Goldschmidt
ISBN 978 1 84819 073 3
eISBN 978 0 85701 048 3

Chair Yoga
Seated Exercises for Health and Wellbeing
Edeltraud Rohnfeld
Illustrated by Edeltraud Rohnfeld
Translated by Anne Oppenheimer
ISBN 978 1 84819 078 8
eISBN 978 0 85701 056 8

Seated Taiji and Qigong
Guided Therapeutic Exercises to Manage Stress and Balance Mind, Body and Spirit
Cynthia W. Quarta
Foreword by Michelle Maloney Vallie
ISBN 978 1 84819 088 7
eISBN 978 0 85701 071 1

COMPLEMENTARY THERAPIES FOR OLDER PEOPLE IN CARE

SHARON TAY

SINGING
DRAGON

LONDON AND PHILADELPHIA

First published in 2014
by Singing Dragon
an imprint of Jessica Kingsley Publishers
73 Collier Street
London N1 9BE, UK
and
400 Market Street, Suite 400
Philadelphia, PA 19106, USA

www.singingdragon.com

Copyright © Sharon Tay 2014

Library of Congress Cataloging in Publication Data
A CIP catalog record for this book is available from the Library of Congress

British Library Cataloguing in Publication Data
A CIP catalogue record for this book is available from the British Library

ISBN 978 1 84819 178 5
eISBN 978 0 85701 141 1

Printed and bound in Great Britain by Bell & Bain Ltd, Glasgow

To all clients who have given me the privilege to serve you and to those who are still with me; I thank you all for giving me the opportunity to share your journey

ACKNOWLEDGEMENTS

Producing this book began 12 years ago. I would like to show appreciation to those who gave their guidance about how to get started in its infant stage: Jean Gilbert, Barbra Tweedie, Carolyn von Opplen and Robin Huygens. Over the years I have appreciated medical advice from Dr Alasdair Diarmid Ross, MBChB, DPH, DTMH, FRACMA, Dr Hugo J. Huygens FRACA, FRCS and Dr Ann Miller MB. MRCP (UK).

During the last three years my support team in assisting me to get this book to publication: Janet Upcher, who through various stages of editing and proofreading and her time dedicated to this project has been exemplary.

To my two colleagues in reflexology, Helen Aldendorff and Chris Line, for proofreading Chapter 7, 'Reflexology and Face Reflexology for Older People in Care'. To Pamela Campbell, for her photography and her patience in preparing the photographs and assisting with the illustrated face charts and foot chart for Chapter 7. Special appreciation goes to Stuart Campbell for computer updates and maintenance and to the photographic models: Angelo Baccarin, Margaret Woods, June Allenby, Catherine Bell and Mrs A. Van Emmerick. Finally, many thanks to Singing Dragon for allowing this book to come to fruition.

CONTENTS

DISCLAIMER

This book is a reference work based on the author's own experience. Any techniques and suggestions are to be used solely at the reader's discretion. The herbal remedies, essential oils and medical treatments described in this book are in no way to be considered as a substitute for consultation with a medical practitioner, and should be used in conjunction with approved medical treatment. The author and publisher are not responsible for any harm or damage to a person, no matter how caused, as a result of following any suggestions in this book.

Introduction

Older people face many challenging changes in their physical and mental well-being when the ageing process accelerates, leaving many frail and elderly persons unable to cater for their own needs. It is during this time that the person becomes more dependent upon the assistance of a relative or health-care worker.

This is one of the most important times in a person's life, the time where the therapist is valuable, bringing to the client many of the services that help to restore dignity and confidence. It should be stated that not all those residing in nursing homes or in other institutions for care are older persons. Some residents are much younger but have ended up in full-time care due to a degenerative illness, accident or disability. Treatments, procedures and safety and hygiene issues dealt with in this book apply equally to such people.

This book is based on my experience from visiting nursing homes, residential homes and hospitals in southern Tasmania. The guidelines presented here may not relate to all nursing homes, therefore it is up to each therapist to follow up specific correct procedures and protocols when visiting any nursing home, aged care or hospice facility. As I state throughout this book, things are constantly changing and each nursing home is different, as is each client.

I have written this book as an introduction for the therapist who intends to treat older and younger persons in care. The book aims to help the therapist to overcome any difficulties that may occur when working with clients. All tips I give have worked well for me over the past 18 years. With constant changes in technology and training, I see a wide scope for therapists working in aged care, especially considering the increasing 'baby boomer' population; there is scope also for work with younger people in care and those in palliative care.

I have gained so much over the years, but I realise there is more to learn and it is up to the therapist constantly to expand their knowledge and explore different techniques while treating frail older persons and young people in care.

As a therapist covering the modalities of beauty therapy, massage therapy, reflexology and naturopathy, a large percentage of my work has involved operating a mobile service. My experience in this field has led me to write this book, as a complement to my first book, *The Carer's Cosmetic Handbook* (Tay 2009). The knowledge and understanding I have gained I wish to pass on to other therapists who may find the information valuable.

In general the people of my generation, the 'baby boomers', are more accepting of complementary therapy treatments than the past generations. The 'baby boomer' generation embraces such therapies as an integral part of everyday health maintenance.

The future holds many possibilities for the therapist, and I can see that there will be an increased need for professionals in the complementary field and other allied heath areas frequently to visit residential homes, hospitals and aged-care facilities. Services will be in much greater demand than before.

Through personal experience, I have come to realise how much these services are needed, although often overlooked. When our senior citizens enter nursing homes, or any other aged care facilities, it does not mean that they should cease to continue with such therapies. It is during this period that a person will benefit most from complementary therapies.

Working in this specialised field is very different from salon or clinic work. It is very challenging, demanding, tiring, sometimes difficult and depressing, and yet it is the most rewarding job any therapist could hope for. It is not a job for the faint-hearted, as there are many issues that may deter a therapist from continuing.

In this book I shall endeavour to cover most topics that relate to the therapist enabling them to learn and understand the protocol and safety issues when treating clients in nursing homes, hospitals or private homes.

It can be disheartening when the client seems to make little or no progress and all the therapist's efforts seem to be in vain. This is often due to the client's general ageing process or to illness and the possibility of side effects from her medication. This is a time when perseverance and dedication are essential. Providing quality care is the most a therapist can do: to do something is much better than doing nothing. In my early professional years, I often felt disappointed that I could not achieve the results I wanted, but continued faithfully in the belief that I might be doing some good. I encourage the therapist not to give up easily. Keep on going and the rewards *will* come. The most important aspect of this work is to give quality care, so that you gain the satisfaction of knowing you have done your best in sometimes difficult circumstances.

For ease of reading I refer to the female throughout the book. This is because it is mainly females that embrace such services. Most of the topics in this book, however, also accommodate male clients.

CHAPTER 1

Support Aids, Special Needs and Communication

PART ONE: SPECIAL AIDS AND SPECIAL NEEDS

The following procedures have been set out covering the topics: special needs: safety and security; communicating with the staff; meeting the client; assessing the client. These procedures encompass my own personal learning, observation and guidelines and are not initiated by any nursing home I have visited. These guidelines have worked successfully over many years, and I continue to follow them.

A VISIT TO A NURSING HOME

The therapist visiting a nursing home will most likely visit a client in her own room. This has advantages for the client:

- comfort in familiar surroundings
- maintainenance of privacy (an important issue)
- problems of mobility resolved.

Possible disadvantage to the therapist is back strain through stooping and bending while treating a client seated in a low chair or lying on a low bed. In the latter years when I have visited the nursing homes in southern Tasmania, I have appreciated the 'upgraded' beds that are better equipped, such as the remote control beds (hospital beds for high care residents) which are easy to operate. Pressing a button can raise the bed to a height suitable for the therapist to work around a client receiving treatment. The head section of the bed can be elevated to sit the client comfortably into a position ready for treatment and both bed ends are removable. The earlier models of these beds have either wind-up or pump levers instead of remote control, but operate in the same manner. Later model beds have made my work a lot easier, as in the past I had to stoop to work at the level of the client's bed. Sixteen years ago, visiting clients residing in aged-care facilities, I found that most residents were able to have their own furniture which included their beds, chairs and other familiar attachments.

Some of the nursing homes I have visited provide a room or a salon where the residents can attend for their treatment, which benefits the operator in the following ways:

- avoids packing and unpacking bags of equipment

- saves time going from room to room

- minimises body stress from bending over low beds and low chairs

- facilitates hygiene practice.

The advantage to clients is that they can enjoy the company of other residents, the social contact and the opportunity to move out of their rooms. Also, I have found these treatment rooms are usually better lit and more spacious than the client's room.

SAFETY AND SECURITY

It is best if the therapist and visitors enter a nursing home or any other aged-care facility by the reception centre so that the office staff will know who they are, and where they will be while on the premises. Also it is a good idea for them to inform the office staff or nursing staff where they will be working and to give an estimate of the time they will be 'in house'. This is mainly a safety measure should the alarm system activate while the therapist is with a client; the staff will then know where to find them. It is most important for a therapist to understand the evacuation procedures for each nursing home, or aged-care facility they visit. For security and identification, I have found it best to wear a name tag so that staff and clients will know who I am. Most nursing homes I have visited have a security system. The allocated areas in the building have a code number, which is used to enter and exit the building. These code numbers may change frequently and therefore a visitor should check with the office staff or a member of the nursing staff in the restricted area. Always keep any code number confidential and never pass it on to any persons in, or outside the premises.

> In the nursing homes I have visited, the office staff have asked me to sign in on arrival and sign out when I leave. This may include noting the client you are visiting and for how long. This is also for safety should the fire alarm activate.

> In Australia it is now required by law that all visiting therapists have a national police search on their profile when working or visiting aged-care facilities, other care homes or when working with children. This applies to employed persons, visiting health care practitioners and volunteers.

COMMUNICATION WITH THE NURSING STAFF

Before making contact with a client in a nursing home, always acknowledge the office staff first, and then go to meet the person in charge who is usually the registered nurse (RN). At times it could be an enrolled nurse or the nurse in charge of the home. Not only is this good relations and courtesy, it is important to find out if there has been any change to the client's well-being since previous visits. The other factor to be considered is the safety and security measures previously mentioned.

When you introduce yourself to the nursing staff mention who made the appointment for your client, especially if this is your first visit. Ask the RN what you need to be aware of regarding your client's condition (see the information and data section in this chapter) and what special needs she may have. If you are not familiar with the client's illness or disability, ask the RN for more information. This applies mostly to a client in high care rather than for a person who is in hostel care (assisted care), which is classified as low care. However, I always make a courtesy visit to the nurses' station when visiting any nursing home. Once you have the information about your client, proceed to the salon in the home or to the client's room. If you are not familiar with the home, ask the RN or another staff member to introduce you to your new client. The nurse or carer will give assistance to the client, if required. If you have visited the client before, a staff member may not be needed unless the client needs assistance.

> Nursing staff will assist the client if she needs to be moved from bed to chair, or into another area. The client may need to be toileted before or during a treatment. She may need help for other reasons that require immediate attention. If a client needs attention while in the middle of their treatment call a carer to assist the client. It is best for the therapist to wait outside the client's room while she is being attended to so that there is more room for the staff to work and for the client's privacy.

After giving the treatment to your client, return to the nurses' station and let the RN know how the client coped with her treatment, and report any concerns about your client that relates to her therapy. If the client is unable to make another appointment and wants to continue to have further treatment, make the appointment with the RN. Staff members who can assist are nursing staff (NS) and the carers, and in some homes I have found a diversional therapist or occupational therapist helpful.

INFORMATION AND DATA

There are a few important questions a therapist may need to ask about her client who is under 'medical care'. This may also apply to hospital patients should a client ask for therapy treatment during their stay. The questions below are some examples that the therapist may find helpful when compiling information. Not all the questions will apply to every client.

- Is the client on any medication that may cause her skin to bruise, show a rash and cause itching, drying or any other skin problems?

- Does she have or has she had any skin cancers, and is she on any medicated creams?

- Does she have any allergy to cosmetics, herbs or essential oils?

- Is she able to see, and does she have any eye problems or eye infections?

- Is she able to communicate and understand instructions?

- How is her hearing?

- How is her mobility?

- (For waxing procedures) ask about her pain threshold.

- Has she had waxing or some form of hair removal previously?

- (For manicure and hand reflexology) does she have any problems related to her fingernails or hands?

  If the client bruises easily, pressure to the skin should be light, and the affected areas should be avoided. Itching can be caused by an irritation or dryness in the skin. If a medication is the cause of the skin condition, the therapist will have an understanding that the skin problems may not heal while the client is taking, or applying medicated creams. A light cosmetic moisture cream or vegetable-based oil may be used if the client is not on any topical medicated cream. Other skin disorders may be treated by a medical person; therefore it is not a good idea to use a cosmetic cream unless given permission. Face waxing may not be an option with frail elderly persons who bruise easily or have a high sensitivity. It is best to avoid any area of the skin that is, or has been, affected by a skin cancer lesion. If the client is on a medicated cream, cosmetic creams may not be suitable. Some clients may be able to use a small amount of a cosmetic cream once the wound has healed and they are no longer on a medicated cream. Face waxing near any cancer lesions should be avoided.

Frail residents residing in a nursing home are often unable to give information on their health. This is where the information session with the nurse is helpful for the therapist. Sometimes this can be difficult. Nursing staff are always busy, especially during administrative work and administering medication. On these occasions I have found it best to arrive a little earlier before the staff become too busy. Another option is to phone the day before and ask for the nurse in charge, to let them know what time you will be in the home to visit the residents. I usually ask for a minute or two of their time in order to catch up on news of my client's progress. When I regularly visit a nursing home, I generally set a time, day and the dates of further visits which are written up on a chart. I leave a copy with the nursing staff so that they will know in advance the days I will be visiting. This method has proved very successful in recent years.

Confidentiality for each resident in a nursing home must be respected. It is not necessary to gather a full medical history, but enough to understand how you need to work with your client, regarding her illness, and what assistance they may need during treatment. Most clients will tell you all about their ailments in detail. If you are unsure about your client's illness or disability, it is best to take the trouble to find out by asking medical staff or by searching through medical textbooks. The internet is a useful tool. It is also a good idea to familiarise yourself with the side effects of any medication a client may be taking, especially medications that may be the cause of problems relating to the skin, fingernails and toenails. Having an understanding of a client's disability or illness can assist the therapist in making improvements to a client's treatment.

THE CLIENT

First impressions are important so, when meeting a client for the first time, be pleasant and speak clearly, so that she will feel at ease. If the person is hard of hearing, the therapist may have to stand in front of the client to get her attention and repeat to the client what has been said. Some hearing impaired persons are able to lip read. However, if the person has a hearing aid, ask her to put in their hearing aid if she has not done so. Stand close, but don't invade her space, just close enough that she can see and hear.

Tell the client what treatment she is going to have. State the procedure, for instance, 'I have come to give you the manicure you have asked for.' Inform her who made the appointment: if it was the client, 'You phoned me yesterday morning asking me to come and give you a manicure,' or, if the appointment was made by a relative or staff member, 'Your daughter phoned to ask me if I would come and visit you, and to give you a manicure, is this okay with you?' The client will either agree or disagree. In some cases I have found that the client cannot remember making any appointment with me and will become confused. If this happens, ask the client if she would like to have treatment. This can be very frustrating, especially if the client does not want to continue with the treatment that had been previously arranged by a relative, nursing staff or by the client. The therapist may find they have come on a wasted journey.

The best method I have found to prevent this from happening is as follows. When a person makes an appointment on behalf of a relative or client who is in care, I make sure I get their details, such as obtaining their name, address and phone number, and who to send the invoice to. I also make it clear that if the treatment is not accepted by the client, and the appointment has not been cancelled before I visit the client, the person making the appointment will be billed for my time and travel. Fortunately most people who make these appointments are reliable for payment. If the appointment is made by staff, ask if the client has a trust fund with the home, or do you send the account to a relative. Never proceed with an appointment unless financial details are finalised.

Before treating a client, assess her first. If all is well, then set up your cosmetics or instruments on a table or bed tray and proceed with her treatment. Always explain to the client what you are going to do, and what benefits the client will gain. Older people like to know what is going on. This gives a sense of security and, more importantly, a say in what they want. Always speak to your clients as you would to a friend, and never speak down to them. Some older people and young people in care have difficulty in communication, but most can understand every word that is being said (see the section on communication, this chapter).

CLIENT ASSESSMENTS AND REPORTS

Assessing the client

To fully assess the client a therapist should observe their mobility and needs after speaking with the RN or other nursing staff. There are specific questions that a therapist may need to ask.

The following list of questions may not relate to every client and the therapist can choose which is relevant.

- Is the client mobile, does she walk with a Zimmer frame or walking stick, or does she need assistance with her wheelchair?

- Does the client use oxygen while having treatment?

- Does the client have any catheters?

- Will the client need medical intervention during treatment (e.g. medication, change tubing, catheters or intravenous feeding)?

- Does the client need to be in a chair or on a bed for her treatment?

- What props do I need to assist the client through treatment (pillows, trays, hand rolls, extra towels, blankets, etc.)?

- Does the client need to have medication, food or water while having treatment? (This can often be an issue with diabetic clients.)

- Will she cope with her treatment?

- Is this a suitable treatment for her?

- Does she understand what is happening?

- Do I need a carer to help lift or prepare my client before treatment?

- Is there a sink with hot and cold water close by?

- Is there an area where I can place my equipment in a safe place?

- Is this a safe and comfortable place for me to work? (Think of the back: will there be too much bending and can I move around the client easily?)

It may be helpful for the therapist to include the following tips in the assessment:

- Consider how to communicate with the client.

- Inspect the skin for any problems, and the texture of the skin.

- Look at the hands and nails and the colour of the nails.

- Observe the skin condition and hair growth that is to be removed by waxing. Is the hair growth coarse, strong, thin or wiry?

Reports

Keeping a record of a client's details is essential, especially if the therapist is not always able to get proper details from the client or from nursing staff. This can happen if the nursing staff are busy or 'short staffed' on the day the therapist visits the home. I have found that writing my observations about the client on the day is very helpful and a good back-up for reference.

The list may include:

- how the client is looking

- if the client is responsive

- if the client is able to have treatment

- if the client wants treatment

- how the client responds to the treatment

- observe the colour of clients skin, nails, lesions, or any changes in these areas since her last treatment

- if the client has changed medication

- if the client has been sick

- if the client is depressed.

The best way to write up a report is to put it in plain English without using technical or medical terms, so that it can be understood by non-medical therapists as well as medical practitioners. A report is a document with valid information to refer to, and should anything arise regarding the client's health and general well-being there will be documentation. It is also a record for the therapist to follow the progress of a client.

> I have always kept a report file on all my clients residing in any aged-care home or residential home and for clients who visit my clinic. Following each visit, I write up the treatment I gave, and any response from the client, either negative or positive, is documented. A report file includes the client's assessment

details as well as the health details that have been passed on by the client, a relative or the RN. It can also include any other relevant details that the therapist may think important. All documents must be kept confidential.

PART TWO: PROSTHESES AND SUPPORT AIDS

Many frail persons rely on some special support equipment or accessories to aid their ability to walk, to sit, to feed, to hear and to see clearly. These include walking frames, wheelchairs and mobile lounge chairs, walking sticks, drinking cups, dentures, hearing aids and glasses. The therapist must be able to work comfortably when treating a client who is reliant on a support aid. It is important to be aware of medical aids such as catheters, colostomy bags and oxygen masks, feeding tubes and other medical equipment when these are being used by a client.

PROSTHESES

A prosthesis is basically an aid that replaces or strengthens a missing or damaged part of the body. The therapist may occasionally come across a person who has lost a limb or limbs; sometimes she may wear the artificial limb, or sometimes not. If the prosthesis is not used, the sleeve or the trouser leg will be folded over the missing limb. Occasionally through the treatment, a client may become a little restless or uncomfortable, and may require extra padding to support the stump of the missing limb. In this case, get nursing staff assistance to attend to the client's needs.

> When I first started out 18 years ago, there were a few clients I came across who had lost a limb or limbs, either through an accident, or through illness such as diabetes. I can remember one client I used to visit regularly who had diabetes. At the beginning of my visits, she was able to walk to her room for treatment. After a year, she lost her right leg and remained in bed for most of the time. Not long after, she lost her other

leg and became very frail. This client still wanted some therapy and was happy for me to give her a facial with face reflexology which helped her to feel relaxed. It gave me satisfaction to know that she had embraced this therapy before she passed away a few months later.

CATHETERS

A catheter is a hollow flexible tube that can be inserted into the body for a variety of reasons:

- administering medications
- administering fluids
- collecting fluids
- monitoring physiological functions
- performing medical procedures.

COLOSTOMY BAGS

A colostomy bag is worn by a person following colon surgery. The two ends of the colon may be brought up to the abdominal surface and sutured (stitched) into place. The opening formed by these two ends is called a stoma. Faecal matter then is eliminated through this opening into a colostomy bag.

If a client is able to have treatment while wearing a catheter or colostomy bag, the therapist must be aware of its location so as not to disturb it in any way. Should a catheter or colostomy bag become dislodged while the client is having her treatment, call for nursing staff right away. Do not wait until treatment is finished.

OXYGEN MASKS

Some people have difficulty breathing on their own and may need to wear an oxygen mask. These fit over the nose and mouth. The mask provides positive airway pressure from an oxygen ventilator during inhalation and exhalation. Some clients are able to have treatment while wearing a mask, for example, during a manicure or hand reflexology.

> In some cases the client can remove the mask from her face for a facial, providing the medical staff have instructed her to do so. It is best for the therapist to check with nursing staff first so they are clear what instructions have been given to the client prior to the therapist's visit.

BRACES

Braces help to support a joint or limb and allow some mobility. Some clients can have therapy while wearing a brace. If the brace can be removed for a short period while they are having treatment the therapist should make sure the support brace is put back on after treatment. Braces can help support the back, neck, arms, legs and knees.

> See nursing staff first and ask if the brace can be removed during the client's treatment. If the client has to keep the brace on, cover the brace with a towel to prevent any cosmetic marks or oil spillage.

DENTURES

Many older people have dentures and some people are inclined to leave them out due to sore gums, gum ulcers or mouth infections. If the client can put in her teeth with comfort, ask her to do so. It is much easier to give a facial wax, or give a facial, when the client has their teeth in. Always let the client or carer handle false teeth. If you have to hand the client's false teeth to her, do so with the teeth in their 'denture' case.

WALKING FRAMES

There are several varieties of walking frames on the market today, some with wheels and some without. The most popular ones that I have seen in the homes are the frames on wheels that have a seat with a basket underneath (often referred to as Zimmer frames). Some clients have used their frames for a seat, hence the term, 'seat walkers'. The person walks with the frame, pushing the frame along and holding on to the handlebars for support. The basket underneath can store her personal things. These frames are light and easy to manoeuvre.

WALKING STICKS

There are some residents in a nursing home or in residential care who will use a walking stick for their support. These walking sticks also come in different colours and sizes. Special walking sticks for visually impaired people are different from the normal walking sticks as they are usually white and fitted with a sound device to aid the person while walking.

WHEELCHAIRS

Fortunately modern wheelchairs are much lighter and easier to push than the older models were. Most of these chairs are fitted with a tray that can be adjusted or taken away. The trays provide useful support when giving a manicure or hand reflexology to a client who is in a wheelchair.

MOTORISED WHEELCHAIRS

These chairs are suitable for clients capable of operating them, as they are registered as limited road vehicles and can be driven on footpaths and side streets. They can be very heavy vehicles; however, their use is perfectly satisfactory by clients during treatment.

MOTORISED OR MOBILITY SCOOTERS

Scooters have been designed for older people to use as vehicles to enable partial independence, in particular for short distances from home. The scooters are similar to motorised wheelchairs in that they travel at a very slow speed and are easy to control. Recently the market has expanded to incorporate various designs of the scooter, and I often see an older person driving one along the footpath when I am out walking in the morning.

MOBILE LOUNGE CHAIRS (RECLINER CHAIRS OR EASY CHAIRS)

A client can lie back more comfortably in this chair. The footrest is adjustable to extend or push back. Again this is a very heavy chair and requires assistance for the client to be wheeled into her room. The advantage of this chair is that the client is comfortable and the practitioner can work around the chair without much difficulty. The disadvantage is that the chair can be low and it can be a strain on the back for the practitioner. Whenever I am treating a client sitting in a lounge chair, I find it helpful to sit on a chair. I have found that these easy chairs are appropriate for treatment of manicures, facial waxes and eyebrow shapes, but not so comfortable for giving a facial or a face massage. The best place I have found for giving facials, massages or foot and face reflexology, is having the client lying in the bed. If it is not practical to have a client transferred to a bed, then work the best you can, but be careful not to put too much pressure on your back or knees while leaning over the chair to the client or bending or stretching.

MOBILE BED TABLES

These movable bed tables are supported on a frame with two extended horizontal bars with wheels. The table can be pushed over the bed for meal times. They can be raised or lowered. Most of these mobile tables are light, and can easily be pushed about in the room. They are useful to place a treatment or cosmetic case upon and for organising equipment.

DRINKING CUPS

Some residents are not very agile with their hands and find things difficult to grasp, especially drinking cups, where spillage is likely. To save the resident from spillage mishaps, cups with lids and straws are often used in these circumstances. Most clients will always have one filled with water, so make sure she has access to their water. The therapist only needs to hand it to her; she is capable of doing the rest. If a client cannot hold a cup she can be assisted by having the cup held up to her mouth while she takes a small sip. If the therapist is not confident to do this, they should ask a carer.

PART THREE: COMMUNICATION AND UNDERSTANDING THE NEEDS OF FRAIL OLDER PEOPLE
MOVING INTO A NURSING HOME

Moving into a new home can be very stressful for most people. When a person has to move into a nursing home, it can be traumatic for her and it can also be a very emotional time. These people are giving up the most valuable gift of all, *independence*. It takes time for many new residents to settle into their new environment, as they are slowly giving away their independence and becoming more reliant on others for their everyday care. They are learning to deal with many changes in routine, getting to know other residents and adjusting to their new rooms, and often sharing with another resident, all of which can be stressful if they are used to being on their own. Most of these residents prefer residing in a single room. Other daily or weekly routines for them include:

- regular meal times

- social outings

- appointments with visiting professionals such as doctors, podiatrists, pharmacists, hairdressers, beauticians, natural therapists and visits from relatives and friends.

Over a period of time most residents do adapt to their new environment and begin to enjoy their new surroundings. They also embrace the attention from external providers and visitors giving them something to look forward to. These residents generally have a positive outlook and accept changes as they come. I have found most of my previous clients have a good sense of humour and are a joy to be with.

The opposite side is when a resident finds difficulty in accepting changes. These people can be difficult, and make life hard for those around them. They are not easy to please and will find fault with many things. Some of these people become fixed in their own world and, no matter what you say or do, things will always remain the same. Some factors which may contribute to a person becoming unsettled are:

- depression

- confusion

- self-centredness (used to being waited on by family and relatives, thus very demanding)

- resentment at being made to go into care

- refusal to accept her illness or disability

- constant pain or trauma.

Sometimes clients in these circumstances will endeavour to gain sympathy, telling the therapist how badly they have been treated by staff or relatives, which can be very distressing for the therapist if they take the story to be 'factual' without realising what the client's 'real' situation is concerning her family and the staff. This is why it is so important for the therapist to have an understanding of what is happening with the client. It is also important for the therapist to show the client that she cares, but not to get involved if the story turns out to be false. Should the client's complaint demonstrate 'factual evidence', the therapist should report the incident/s to the person in charge of the home and document it in the client's report file. In my experience, I have found that though a client is initially distressed with the many challenges she has to face, she eventually adapts and, by the time I visit her again, she is more settled and happy. It is not surprising that these are the clients who will want to have therapy treatments. Over time, when they get used to their new environment and make friends with the other residents, many begin to enjoy the social side offered by the nursing home and they participate in the daily activities as well as looking forward to regular visits from a therapist or visitor.

> For four years I visited a woman in a nursing home on a regular fortnightly basis. She was a client who had difficulty in accepting her new home and constantly complained about the staff. The staff were very good and helpful and tried all the time to encourage her to go out on the residents' bus for afternoon tours with the other residents, and attend in-home entertainment, which she often refused. She was always well attended, showered and put into her bed by the time I arrived at 9.30am to give her treatment. She felt she was neglected and nobody cared. Her conversation was the same over the four years that I knew her. I knew off by heart what she was going to say, and sometimes, when my energy was low, I could have walked out on her. However, over time, when she finally accepted me, and I became familiar with her ongoing complaints, I realised what her 'real' problem was, and I could see why she was unhappy. This woman did not want to live in a nursing home. She was hard to please but, strangely, she loved her treatment and always greeted me with a smile. However, if I was sick, or if I went on a holiday, she did not greet me so well when I returned, and would scold me for not coming to visit her. (I knew for sure she was missing my visits.) No matter what

I said, I could not convince her that I too, needed a break. She had a habit of asking me how I was and, before I could answer, she would go into her own world and constantly talk about herself. This was one self-absorbed person. Over the years I did grow fond of her, and I came to appreciate the experience I had gained by persevering with this woman. She was a 'great' teacher in many ways and I had learned many things through her, especially with patience and understanding. Thank you, Mrs B.

DEALING WITH DEMENTIA

Dementia is the 'umbrella' term used for a large group of illnesses, including Alzheimer's disease, which cause progressive decline in a person's mental functioning, such as a loss of memory, intellect, rationality, social skills and normal emotional reactions. There are various types of dementia, but Alzheimer's disease is one of the most common types. The effects of different types of dementia are similar, but not identical, as each one tends to affect different parts of the brain (Bryden 2005, p.183).

Over the years, treating older persons with beauty therapy and reflexology, I have found a large percentage of clients have some form of forgetfulness, or dementia. Treating clients with memory loss is certainly not a deterrent for the therapist. In my experience, I have found most clients with dementia embrace the comfort of 'touch': the comforting tactile aspects of treatments and the attention given to them. Depending on the nature of their memory loss, some clients can become very confused by simple instructions. A therapist needs to be very patient and understanding and constantly let the client know what is happening. Clients with advanced memory loss cannot remember what day it is, or what they did five minutes ago. They will often ask a question and, by the time a therapist has answered it, they will ask it again, and this can continue throughout the treatment. Confusion is very difficult for the client as well as it is for her carer or therapist, who both need to have a good sense of humour, and plenty of time and energy, because working with such clients can be very exhausting and, at times, frustrating. There are many problems associated with people who suffer from some form of dementia. Confusion is first on the list: I have witnessed this when a client had put away her things, and later not remembered where she had put them. When this happened, the client became very agitated, and accused someone of stealing. I told her that I saw her put them in the corner on the table. She argued that this could not possibly be so, as she knew they were stolen. I could see that this might lead to an argument. I managed to direct her to sit in her chair to have her usual manicure. When she sat down she could see the cosmetics set up before her on a table and then she looked at me for the first time and said, 'Oh, you are the lady who comes to do my nails. I did not see you come in I am so glad you are here.' This is one scenario and there are many more.

Clients with dementia will often misplace things and can never remember where they have put them: this leads to anxiety and agitation causing the client to become more unsettled. In a nursing home a resident may often lose money or their personal belongings, mostly through putting them in a 'safe place' and forgetting where they have put them. Unfortunately, things can go missing, and sometimes they can later be found, or perhaps not. Fellow residents affected by dementia may take things, believing them to be their own. A further problem for residents may be the loss of clothing misplaced in the establishment's laundry. A few of my clients have told me that they have seen another resident wearing their clothes. Labelling of clothing does not necessarily prevent this problem from happening. If your client complains about missing money or personal belongings, advise them to speak to the nursing staff. The therapist can mention it to the RN if they feel that there is a genuine concern.

No matter what the client's memory loss, if she wants your services, persevere, as this is one of the most fulfilling experiences a therapist may gain. The therapist will develop in communication skills and in the ability to handle difficult situations. (For more on dementia refer to Chapter 2, 'Medication, Illness and Nutritional Impairments'.)

Older people from their 70s onwards will often refer to the nursing staff as 'sister', 'matron' or 'nurse' (the carer). This is because they only remember the old system of hospital training up until the mid-1980s (in Tasmania), when nursing staff were addressed more formally.

PRIVACY ISSUES

It is very important that clients have privacy when receiving their treatment, especially for those who are visually impaired. Do not let them be exposed to other people about them, even if it is only for a manicure. Allow them their dignity. Ask the carer or a nurse to take them to their room, so that they can have their 'special time' with you. If the client is sharing a room with another resident, draw a curtain around the bed so that the client can feel comfortable without other prying eyes. Remember, residents are constantly exposed to a lot of people, especially in a nursing home, and all the comings and goings of people in the place. Therefore, some quiet time alone is very important for them.

When I visit a client in their room, I always place a Do Not Disturb sign outside the door. This is so visitors cannot interrupt, and so nursing staff can know where I am if I am needed or if there should be a fire alarm. This sign does not exclude nursing staff if they have to come into the room and give the client her medication or some other medical procedure. If the therapist is working from a salon that is situated in a nursing home, most mobile clients are happy to share their time in the company of other residents while they are having their treatment, so there is no need to put a Do Not Disturb sign on the door. You can indicate that the therapist is at work in the salon by setting up a workplace, and putting a sign outside the door to let passing residents know the therapist is in the salon and available for customers. The carer or the RN will often let residents know the days the therapist will visit the home, providing the therapist has left a list of dates and times of visits.

EMPATHY AND SYMPATHY

The difference between empathy and sympathy is that *empathy* is the sharing of another's feelings, the ability to share an emotion, sensation or condition. It is the capacity to be more involved emotionally and to take on the sharing of a problem. *Sympathy* is the ability to identify with a person or object: to understand, care, but not take on board another person's problems.

When working in a nursing home or visiting older persons in their homes, the therapist will see her client's environment, and possibly hear from the client or her carer, or a relative, the difficulties the client has to face each day. This can be very distressing to witness and hear and, as a professional, the therapist must not get involved on the emotional level, but at the same time she can be 'understanding' and caring towards her client's suffering. This is sympathy. You have to learn to walk away and leave the problem where it is.

If you feel the client is in danger, then, and only then, should you contact someone who can help them. Some clients through their loneliness will talk of being neglected by family and friends, and so on. This is not always the case, as often family members are doing more than their share of being there to cater for the client's needs. This is why it is important for the therapist to be skilled in dealing with emotional upsets and understanding their client's situation.

DETACHMENT (FOR THE THERAPIST)

It is very important that you leave your work and not dwell on the bad things you may have seen, or have dealt with, through the day. You are no use to your other clients if you are carrying any load from a previous client, as this can interfere with your work. If you are having difficulty in detaching from the problem, talk to a friend or colleague who can be a good listener. If it is a client you are worried about, pass it on to the nursing staff or a relative if the client's problem is presenting any danger. It is not your problem.

DEATH OF A CLIENT

Sadly, the reality is that older residents in nursing homes and in palliative care are at the last stage of their lives, and only 'time' can determine when God will come to take them home. You cannot guarantee how long you will have these clients on your books. This is why it is important that you give the best of your care, and enjoy every visit, giving full attention and time to the treatment that they like to have.

The death of a client can sometimes be a sad experience, especially if there has been a special 'bond' shared over a long period. Dealing with the death of a client is not pleasant but, with experience, the therapist will learn to cope and accept that her responsibility is to the living, and it is to the living that she must give her full attention. Sometimes the nursing home staff may inform the therapist about her client's passing before her next visit, other times the therapist will turn up and be told. This is not being harsh, it is a way of life, and the nursing staff are used to seeing it all the time and would appreciate that a therapist accepts the passing of a client in the same manner. This does come with experience.

In my experience, I have found many clients were happy to face their final days in life and are realistic about what little time they may have left. Some women will often state that they have come to this home to live out their last days, or that they haven't got long to live. When you are faced with these statements, do not tell a client that she is being silly, or that she has plenty of years ahead of her, or some other unrealistic remark, as this only demeans her coming to terms with the inevitable. The best you can do is to acknowledge her remarks by just listening. Some clients will only make a statement, while others may like to talk about it. I have also been asked by a few clients, whether I believe there is a God. The only way I have been able to answer this question without having to project my personal beliefs, or interfere with the client's personal beliefs is to answer as follows: 'I do believe that there is a wonderful being who creates us and takes us, and that everything has a reason, even though you and I may never understand why.'

COMMUNICATION IMPAIRMENT

Making conversation can sometimes be difficult for the client, especially if her speech is impaired. This is where communication skills come to the test. For example, people who have suffered a stroke will often have difficulty with speech.

After a period of time, some sufferers will regain their speech, while others do not. Speech can be slow or slurred, and this is when the therapist will need a lot of patience to understand what the person is trying to say.

Other factors that may relate to poor communication are:

- loss of speech

- English may not be the native language

- hearing difficulties

- sore gums or tongue

- depression

- dementia.

The important issue here is for the therapist to help the client make conversation, but not to take over and sound like a 'talking parrot'. This can be annoying for the client. The therapist should just make pleasant conversation with short sentences and allow the client time to respond. If the client does not want to respond or cannot, just work quietly through touch and care. Remember, the client may just want to have her treatment in peace and quiet, especially if she is in her own room. Read her body language.

When a client is ready to talk, encourage her to do so by listening and let her know that you have understood what she has said. It is amazing how quickly the therapist can become familiar with a client's 'impaired' words and sentences, when she has taken the time to listen and give extra quality of care to her client. I have found this to be very rewarding when a client can feel comfortable in communication and knowing that I have understood what she was saying. A good relationship between a therapist and a client will encourage the client to continue with her therapy treatments, and both will look forward to regular visits.

> For 13 years I had visited a client in her mid-50s who had had a stroke, residing in a nursing home. She also had Type 2 diabetes and was overweight due to the medication she was taking. When I first met her in 1996, I really had difficulty in trying to work out what she was telling me, and didn't know how I was to communicate with her. My client was unable to write, although she was able to understand every word I said, so writing notes was not an option. One day while I was giving her a manicure, she kept talking. I realised she was asking me something, as she kept repeating the same sentence, and I could see her getting agitated because I was not responding. I stopped what I was doing, held her hand, and asked her to forgive me. I said, 'I have difficulty in hearing sometimes and please be patient with me, speak slowly, and let me repeat after you, and would you nod your head if I have understood what you had said.' It took me a long time to work from this method, but over time I was able to recognise many of her sentences and words, and because of this, we formed a wonderful therapist to client relationship. We both enjoyed our 'quality' time with laughter, good stories to tell, and my client always looked forward to our 'girlie chats' and her beauty treatment. I began to apply this same method to all clients I was treating, especially when I started out in my 'novice' years. When I approached a disabled client for the first time, I always asked them if they could teach me how they liked to be handled, and what I needed to do to help make them feel comfortable. This was the only way I could learn, and it

was also empowering for them, because they had a say in what they wanted. It is important to allow a person in care to have their 'rights' in what they want. Many people mean well, but will often talk down to a frail older person or a disabled person, disempowering them and making them feel vulnerable and completely dependent.

Always let a client do the things they can do for themselves; just be there to give her support should she need your assistance. When walking with a client who is visually impaired, let her hold your arm, and walk with her, do not pull her along. Explain clearly where you are going, and guide her gently to where she needs to go. If you are giving treatment to a visually impaired person in her room, make sure the 'things' you move are put back in the same position where you had found them when you entered the room.

CHAPTER 2

Medication, Illness and Nutritional Impairment

PART ONE: MEDICATION AND ITS SIDE EFFECTS

The majority of older people and those in palliative care are on prescribed medication. Long-term medication can have side effects which subsequently lead to poor nutrition. The effects of medication can also contribute to skin disorders, facial hair problems (excess facial hair or loss of hair), and medication can affect the normal growth in the fingernails and toenails.

SIDE EFFECTS TO THE SKIN

Poor circulation. The signs may be:

- the skin can feel cold, especially in the feet, hands and fingers

- the skin may look pale or pinkish and the client can be sensitive to cold weather

- numbness in the hands or feet, or both

- the skin may also appear with a bluish hue, especially around the lips.

Other problems that may occur in the skin are:

- the accumulation of dead skin cells in specific areas such as the head, around the eyes, on top of the forehead, lower and upper arms, lower and upper part of legs

- bruising

- dry skin

- skin thinning

- loss of pigmentation in the skin and hair

- discolouration of the skin

- slow wound healing

- cracking or deep furrowing in the feet, and fingers and the lips, which are not uncommon areas to be affected.

Other visible signs are:

- swelling in the face, hands and feet

- skin rashes such as hives

- sore eyes.

SIDE EFFECTS TO THE FINGERNAILS AND TOENAILS

Nail abnormalities often result from nutritional deficiencies, infections, illness, injury, or improper manicure or pedicure procedures. The following are some of the disorders I have found in some of my frail clients:

- thickening of the nails

- brittle nails

- splitting in nails

- ridges

- white spots

- discolouration

- nail shedding

- soft thin nails

- blue nails

- large wide nails

- excess of dead skin under nails

- cuticle disorders.

(See more on fingernail problems in Chapter 4.)

UNWANTED FACIAL HAIR GROWTH

Excess facial hair growth needs regular attention, as hair continuously grows, and it can either become very soft or very coarse and wiry. Coarse facial hair that is removed by shaving, hair removal creams and by careless tweezing may also create problems in the skin such as:

- pustules

- ingrown hair

- clogged pores

- scarring

- skin-piercing

- papules.

Eyebrows can grow in different directions on older people. They can become very wiry and strong, showing white or grey thick strands, or they can thin out into fine strands. On some women there are no visible eyebrow hairs at all. Clients will often ask why these problems happen. Explain to them how they may be caused and how you may be able to improve them.

The skill of the therapist is to be confident, showing the client she can give her special care, helping to improve her fingernails or skin complaint, but the treatments may not give the results the client had hoped for. In my experience I have found that women who have beauty treatments or natural therapy treatments regularly can achieve satisfactory results, even though they know they will never have the healthy fingernails or skin that preceded their illness. The focus is to give quality of care, and special individual attention.

> In cases of illness or medication, clients can often give you full details of their illness and their medication and I have found this to be a great help. Through my clients I have learned a lot over the years and, together with the help of medical textbooks and research on the internet, my clients have helped me to learn and to clear any 'misunderstandings' I may have had.

PART TWO: ILLNESS AND DISABILITIES

Multiple illnesses and disabilities are common among older people and for younger persons in care. Not only is beauty therapy and hairdressing a 'look and feel good' enhancement, natural therapies have also been known to alleviate or soothe many ailments, especially helping to induce relaxation and sleep, and helping in improving fingernail care and some minor skin disorders. I will mention a few of these therapies, and those I have used over the years. Many of my clients have found them to be effective.

(See more on natural therapies in Chapter 6 and reflexology in Chapter 7.)

> Medical permission must be approved before using any natural therapy on a frail person. Some herbal or essential oils may be contraindicated with certain medications. People with a sensitivity and an intolerance to strong fragrant odours may react to the smells in some essential oils and herbs. They may not tolerate these applications.

DEMENTIA AND ALZHEIMER'S DISEASE

Dementia is not a disease, but an 'umbrella' term for a variety of symptoms that may accompany or indicate certain diseases or conditions. Today over 60 different conditions are known to cause dementia symptoms. Symptoms may include impaired memory and confusion, difficulty in performing day-to-day or familiar tasks, and changes in personality, mood and behaviour. When caused by disease or injury, dementia is usually irreversible, however, the symptoms may be reversible when caused by treatable conditions, such as dehydration, constipation, infection, vitamin deficiencies and imbalances, pain, medication poisoning, brain tumours or depression (Verity 2009).

Alzheimer's disease is one of the most common causes of dementia. It is a result of damage and changes to nerve cells within the brain. It causes cognitive, emotional and personality changes. As the disease progresses, these changes become more severe. The therapist needs to be very patient and understanding when treating a client with dementia. It is best not ask too many questions at a time. People who suffer with memory loss can only deal with short questions and simple instructions that may have to be repeated several times. There are some rules that the therapist must be aware of when treating people with dementia, and this should also apply to all frail older persons and to young people in care. They are:

- Always respect the client and never speak down to her: it is degrading and unprofessional.

- Never speak about the client in front of her. When you greet your client, tell her who you are, and then ask her if she wants to have her treatment.

- Keep the client's appointment short: longer sessions may tire her. Some clients with dementia can easily become agitated and restless during longer sessions.

BEAUTY THERAPY FOR CLIENTS WITH DEMENTIA

In my experience most clients who suffer with dementia are able to cope with their beauty treatment and embrace the service. Some clients may not always remember the dates or times for their appointments, but some have recognised me by my cosmetic bag. I have found that a few clients may take longer to become familiar with what was happening, until they see the cosmetics in front of them on a bed tray or table, and then they can remember who I am. It is important for the therapist to help the client feel relaxed and allow her to enjoy her therapy without too many distractions. I have found that some clients can become restless and stressed if there are people coming in and out of their rooms while they are having their treatment. This was a big issue in my early years. I found it was best to place a Do Not Disturb sign on the door. Most visitors will respect a resident's privacy.

When applying skin care products, use minimal cosmetics and keep the applications basic. Lately, I have stopped applying lipstick to some frail older women due to the problems they have with their lips, teeth, gums and ingesting lipsticks through involuntary lip movements and by sucking on their lips.

HAIRDRESSING

Hairdressing is essential for older people, especially women. Many look forward to the weekly service offered by the home, while others may visit a hairdressing salon near the nursing home. Most nursing homes I have visited have a hairdresser who attends to the residents regularly. The homes provide a salon or a special room the hairdresser can use. I have noticed that many of my clients who have dementia will remember having their hair done although they may not remember when. I can understand why older people like to have their hair done. Not only does it make them feel good after the treatment, but the soothing head massage encourages relaxation when their hair is being washed. This also helps to relax a restless client.

> Many a time I have been mistaken for the hairdresser by some of my clients. I let them know that I am not the hairdresser, I am the beautician or reflexologist. They accept this, but on a few occasions they have asked me to do their hair after having their beauty treatment. I make it clear to them that I am not able to do their hair like the hairdresser; I can only comb it for them. I realise that the motion of the comb or the brush going through their hair makes them feel more relaxed. They tell me I

have done a wonderful job and they would be so lost if I did not come to do their hair.

This is typical of clients with dementia. As much as they enjoy having therapy treatments, they can become confused about which therapy they are having.

NATURAL THERAPIES FOR RESIDENTS IN AGED CARE

During my time as a beauty therapist treating older clients, I have also incorporated natural therapies that have included aromatherapy, herbal applications, massage, colour therapy and reflexology, especially face and hand reflexology. There are many other alternative therapies that are possibly compatible with illnesses or disorders of the eyes or skin listed below, but I will mention those that I have practised and others that I have known to help. Although I do not teach Tai Chi, I have found it to be a very good therapy for my arthritis and I have seen residents in a nursing home enjoy a session of Tai Chi with the occupational therapist or a Tai Chi instructor. Music therapy has also been known to help calm many an agitated resident, especially if it is music with which she is familiar. In fact, I have found some of the music being played to residents while I am treating a client to be very soothing and relaxing, especially 'old time' tunes ranging from the decades of the 1920s through to the 1960s. Familiar music will often motivate a resident to sing along with the tune. It is also encouraging to see performing artists visit the homes and entertain the residents. Many enjoy the sing-along.

PARKINSON'S DISEASE (PD)

Parkinson's disease is a neurological illness named after Dr James Parkinson, a London physician who was the first to describe it in 1817. PD is a disorder caused by the gradual loss of cells in a small part of the brain called the *substantia nigra*. The death of these cells produces a reduction in a vital chemical called dopamine, which causes symptoms that may include:

- shaking of hands
- slowing down of movement
- stiffness
- loss of balance
- loss of facial expression
- speech impairment
- difficulty swallowing
- handwriting difficulties
- urinary problems
- constipation
- dry skin
- depression.

Parkinson's disease is a progressive disorder, and these symptoms worsen with time (Parkinson's Study Group 2009).

Beauty therapy tips for people with Parkinson's disease

Clients with PD can enjoy beauty therapy, especially a manicure or a facial. When giving a manicure, if the client is seated in a chair, the therapist can put a pillow or cushions covered with a clean towel over the client's lap and have her rest her hands on top of the pillow. If the client's tremors are severe, roll up a hand towel or face flannel (resembling a sausage) and place the client's hands over the towelling roll. This helps to settle the tremors. Hold each finger firm and file the fingernails. Do not use any scissors for cutting the fingernails if the client's tremors are severe.

Do not use nail varnish with PD clients as the strong fumes can be overpowering for most.

Natural therapy tips for the therapist

I have found that, when I treat PD clients, their tremors settle when I give them head and face reflexology. The clients relax and enjoy the therapy. When I give a manicure, I incorporate hand reflexology that helps to settle the shaking in the client's hands. Do not use strong fragrant oils as they can cause the person to become more agitated. I have seen this happen and the client's tremors can become worse, especially when the oils have been placed in front of her or applied to her skin.

> Sweet almond oil and calendula oils have proved to be reasonably safe when treating older persons irrespective of their illness or skin disorder. However, always patch test a client before using any essential oils.

CARDIOVASCULAR DISEASE

The term cardiovascular disease (CVD) refers to any heart and blood vessel disease, including high blood pressure, stroke, heart failure, peripheral vascular disease (which often occurs in older people, mostly affecting lower limbs) and deep vein thrombosis (DVT).

Heart disease

Heart disease is any disorder that affects the heart's normal functioning. The condition is a chronic one affecting both genders. The coronary arteries (those that supply the heart muscle with oxygen) become clogged with 'plaque', a fatty substance. Plaque accumulates gradually on the inner lining of the arteries, narrowing them. This is called atherosclerosis, and basically means the blood supply to the heart muscle is reduced due to narrowing of the arteries, which often leads to angina. In the narrowed artery a clot of blood forms, blocking supply of blood to parts of the heart. This can cause a heart attack.

Beauty and reflexology tips for clients with a heart disorder

The lunula in the fingernails can show a pink to reddish hue in clients with heart disorders including high blood pressure. The nails can be either thick, or thin. However, with some clients the nails have a tendency to chip, fray and remain short. Careful consideration must be given when giving a manicure. Do not use nail varnish. (See more on caring for the nails in Chapter 4.)

CEREBROVASCULAR DISEASE (CD) (STROKE)

CD or a stroke occurs when the supply of blood to the brain is suddenly disrupted. Blood is carried to the brain by blood vessels called arteries. Blood may stop moving through an artery because the artery is blocked by a blood clot or plaque, or because the artery breaks or bursts.

A stroke is not just an 'old age' disease, it can happen to anyone at any time. The way in which people are affected by stroke depends where in the brain the stroke occurs and the size of the stroke. For example, someone who has a minor stroke may only be affected with a few side effects. On the other hand, someone who has a major stroke may be left totally paralysed on one side, or in a coma, or may die due to the extent of the stroke (Stroke Foundation 2007).

Important tips for the therapist

A person may be on anticoagulants (a range of medicines including aspirin) to help prevent blood clots. Should a client be on any blood-thinning medication and she bleeds, it can take longer for her wound to stop bleeding and heal. This is why it is important for the therapist to know this, because of the nature of waxing procedures and some manicure procedures, especially if the client has thin skin. Besides treating many clients with dementia, I have also treated a number of stroke sufferers who can experience dementia. Some clients have been as young as 39. Most of the clients I have treated ranged from 50 through to their 80s.

Beauty therapy and hand reflexology tips for stroke clients

To give a manicure use the 'roll' towel to place in the affected hand with the fingers coming over top of the roll this will help to relax any trembling. If the affected hand cannot be immersed in a bowl of warm water for soaking, use a warm wet towel that has been soaked in water with an antibacterial solution. Make sure the hand and skin between the fingers are washed and dried thoroughly. The hand can become infected with a fungal or a bacterial infection through careless hygiene procedures if it is not properly cared for. Leaving the hand moist without regular cleansing is a common cause of infections. The fingernails on the affected hand may be very weak, with the fingernail curving over the nail pad on the finger. The nail may look white, and if the lunula is absent it may be a sign of anaemia or malnutrition. I have observed that the skin on stroke sufferers can be very dry and often scaly. Their sensitivity can be very high and some women may not be able to cope with any form of waxing procedures although most others can. This is why it is always important to patch test on clients with skin disorders and ill health.

Natural therapy tips for stroke clients

Many of my clients who have had a stroke can cope with some natural therapies such as massage, aromatherapy and, especially, face reflexology. I have found that many clients relax, and they tell me they feel 'so good' after the treatment. Most like having their face touched. I have seen a few clients react with a 'high' sensitivity showing a bright red colour to their skin from strong fragrant aromatherapy oils, so it is best to keep it simple and only use a base oil like sweet almond, which has proved suitable for most people.

ARTHRITIS

Arthritis is often referred to as a single disease. In fact, it is an 'umbrella' term for many medical conditions that affect the musculoskeletal system, specifically joints where two or more bones meet. While there are about 100 forms of arthritis, the three most significant are:

- osteoarthritis

- rheumatoid arthritis

- gout.

Besides these three, there are other common forms of arthritis:

- ankylosing spondylitis

- juvenile arthritis

- systemic lupus erythematosus (lupus)

- scleroderma.

(Better Health Channel 2013a)

Osteoarthritis commonly develops from the age of 45, although it can occur in younger people. Many people have symptoms as they age, such as stiffness, joint pain and muscle weakness. Osteoarthritis has a reputation of being a disabling disease. While some people suffer from constant pain, others are only troubled by joint stiffness from time to time. The areas that are most affected are:

- the hands – usually the end finger joints

- the spine – in the neck and lower spine

- hips – older people are most at risk

- knees – may be caused by an old injury.

(Better Health Channel 2013d)

Rheumatoid arthritis is a chronic disease, mainly characterised by inflammation of the lining, or synovium of the joints. It can lead to long-term joint damage, resulting in chronic pain, loss of function and disability. It is the second most common arthritis after osteoarthritis (Healthinsite 2008).

Gout is a common form of arthritis caused by the build-up of a waste product, uric acid, in the bloodstream. Normally uric acid is dissolved in the bloodstream and filtered out by the kidneys and excreted in urine. Build-up of uric acid may settle in the joints in the form of crystals, causing inflammation and pain. This is called gout. The joint of the big toe is the first site to be affected; it becomes red and swollen and can be extremely painful. The other areas to be affected are the joints of all the toes, knees and ankle (Better Health Channel 2013b).

As an arthritis sufferer myself, I find it is very hard to get started in the morning as it can take a few minutes before I can manoeuvre myself from a lying position into a sitting position and move up to a standing position. This is because my knee joints, legs and back are painful and stiff. I am most seriously affected with stiffness and pain on very cold days or on very hot days. I can empathise with many of my clients who suffer from some form of arthritis. What most arthritis sufferers have in common is that they can feel very tender on any part of their body when they are being touched, especially when they are in pain. When the joints are affected they can become swollen and, in some people, they can become disjointed especially in the finger joints making the hands look enlarged and disabled. The fingernails have a tendency to dry out and the nail plate can become either hard or brittle with furrows, and the free-edge of the nail tends to split and fray. The skin has a tendency to become dehydrated and, because of this, itching is common among those who have a dry or dehydrated skin. Itching also leads to inflammation and rashes if left unattended. Tiredness, exhaustion and depression are common symptoms associated with arthritis sufferers. Because of all the underlying problems that go with arthritis, it is best for the therapist to work carefully when treating the skin, hands and fingernails of a person with arthritis.

Natural therapies for arthritis sufferers

I have found foot reflexology beneficial for my pain. Other therapies that have helped arthritis sufferers are exercise, Tai Chi, acupuncture or acupressure. I do not think acupuncture would be advisable for frail older persons, but a few of my clients, colleagues and friends have said that they have had acupuncture and found it helped, whereas others said it did not help them. Like Western medicine, not all natural therapies will benefit everyone. It is a matter for the individual to find what suits her best, and how she responds to a therapy.

LUPUS

Lupus is an autoimmune disease where the body's immune system becomes hyperactive and attacks normal, healthy tissue. This results in symptoms such as inflammation, swelling, and damage to joints, skin, kidneys, blood, the heart and lungs. This is known as systemic lupus erythematosus (SLE). There are several kinds of lupus. Discoid lupus is limited to the skin.

People with lupus suffer many symptoms, including:

- pain and swelling of joints
- muscle pain
- fever
- red rash on the face
- chest pain when taking a breath

- hair loss

- pale or purple fingers or toes

- sensitivity to the sun

- mouth ulcers

- fatigue

- swollen glands.

Other symptoms may include:

- anaemia

- headaches

- depression

- confusion

- seizures.

Symptoms may come and go ranging from mild to severe and when a person is having any of the above number of symptoms these periods are referred to as 'flares'.

MULTIPLE SCLEROSIS (MS)

Multiple sclerosis is the most common chronic disease of the central nervous system among young Australians. First symptoms appear in young adults between 20 and 50 years. It mostly affects people of Caucasian origin and 70 per cent of people affected are females. MS occurs when the protective sheath (myelin) around the nerve fibres in the brain and spinal cord becomes damaged, causing random patches called plaques or lesions. These patches distort and interrupt the messages that are sent along these nerves. 'Sclerosis' means scar and the disease is labelled 'multiple' because the damage usually occurs at a number of points.

The health effects of this disease are varied and no two people will share the same symptoms. The cause of MS is unknown and, as yet, there is no cure. However, treatments are available to ease the symptoms and modify the course of the disease. Some people with MS may become seriously disabled. Others may have one or two attacks and then remain symptom-free for the rest of their lives (Better Health Channel 2013c).

Tips for treating a client with MS

The therapist should be aware that sufferers during a relapse, or at the later stages of the disease, can become very exhausted and tired, especially on hot days. Also, each individual can respond differently with their senses, especially to touch, and some sufferers may feel tender or sore during a treatment. Speech can also be affected and may become more slurred when the individual feels tired or exhausted. There are certain times of the day when a client may not be able to have a treatment, especially if it is a hot day. The therapists must be prepared to change an appointment for the client, and arrange a time that is suitable for both. I have found it is much easier for the client and the therapist (less back strain) if the client can have their treatment lying in bed, especially if the client is feeling tired and exhausted. Some people with MS may not have the 'noticeable' symptoms mentioned – it could be that they are not experiencing such a 'severe patch' as those who are suffering with the illness at its worst. The treatment the therapist gives the client may vary from a full-time session to a short session, depending on how the client is coping. It is important not to exhaust, or 'over-service', the client. Clients with MS will need to be treated carefully due to their sensitivity.

> When I was introduced to my first client in 1994, she had severe MS and was physically disabled and speech impaired. She was in her late 40s. This was a challenge for a 'novice' therapist, as I had never come across anyone with MS and especially in the advanced stage of this woman. By trial and error, and with patience, I finally found a way that made her feel comfortable during her treatments and discovered the best way for me to

be able to move about with ease. The biggest hurdle I had to overcome was with her fingernails. Because of her illness and the medication she was taking, her nails were in very poor condition. She was prone to suffer with psoriasis in the nails and this would often lead to a fungal infection. The nails were very brittle and white, and underneath the nails the psoriasis looked yellow and resembled fine crumbs. Holding her hands could sometimes prove to be very painful for her. This became a dilemma at times as I was unfamiliar with how to deal with such problems. However, over time and with research and experience, I was able to find a way that she could feel relaxed when I gave her a manicure. Using the essential oil mixture proved to be successful in removing dirt and improving the fingernails.

(See the section on 'Over-servicing' in Chapter 9, 'The Code of Ethics and the Delicate Balance'.)

DIABETES

Diabetes is a chronic disease that is life-lasting. For our bodies to function properly we need to convert glucose from food to energy. The hormone insulin is essential for the conversion of glucose into energy. For people with diabetes, insulin is no longer produced or not produced in sufficient amounts in the body. Foods such as breads, cereals, fruit and starchy vegetables, legumes, milk, yoghurt and sweets, can't be converted into energy by people who have diabetes. The glucose stays in the blood making the glucose levels higher. There are several types of diabetes:

- Type 1 diabetes
- Type 2 diabetes
- gestational diabetes
- hypoglycaemia

- hyperglycaemia

- ketoacidosis.

Type 1 diabetes

The pancreas stops making insulin, and the body cells cannot turn glucose into energy. Without insulin the body burns its own fats as a substitute. Insulin must be given daily to prevent dangerous chemical substances in the blood resulting from the burning of fat. This can cause a condition known as ketoacidosis, which is potentially life-threatening if not treated.

The symptoms of ketoacidosis show high blood glucose levels and moderate ketones in the urine with:

- rapid breathing

- flushed cheeks

- abdominal pain

- sweet acetone (similar to paint thinner or nail polish) smell on the breath

- vomiting

- dehydration.

(Diabetes Australia 2009)

In my experience I have only dealt with a few clients with Type 1 diabetes and they have been younger women. I have found their skin to be very dry, scaly, flushed and their nails to be very white with reddish hues and some fingernails had yellow spots. The fingernails can also be thin and frail. Waxing procedures have proved to be too painful and it is not a good idea for some women to have waxing as they can be at a higher risk for infections. Infections are difficult to clear as healing is very slow and this can lead to other complications for people with diabetes.

Type 2 diabetes

This is the most common form of diabetes, mostly affecting older persons. However, recently more and more young people are getting Type 2 diabetes, even children. In Type 2 diabetes the pancreas makes some insulin but it is not produced in the amount the body needs and it does not work effectively. Type 2 diabetes results from a combination of genetic and environmental factors. Besides a genetic link, other factors that can lead to Type 2 diabetes are:

- high blood pressure

- overweight or obesity

- insufficient physical activity

- poor diet

- the classic 'apple'-shape body, where weight is carried around the waist.

Type 2 diabetes can be managed with healthy eating and exercise. Over time most people will need to manage their diabetes with tablets and many will need insulin.

A person with symptoms for Type 2 diabetes may show:

- excessive thirst

- frequent urination during the day

- feeling tired and exhausted

- experiencing constant hunger

- slow healing of wounds

- itching and skin infections

- weight gain

- mood swings

- headaches

- leg cramps

- feelings of dizziness.

(Diabetes Australia 2009)

I have come across many clients in care who have Type 2 diabetes. Many have very similar symptoms to Type 1 diabetes, showing dry and scaly skin. Some clients have a flushed face and their hands can also be red. I have found using the essential nail oils very good, helping to combat infections and improving peeling skin around the nail (another common problem with dry nails and skin). Some women can cope with waxing procedures, but it is best to use cold wax strips and not hot wax.

> I can remember one woman I used to visit regularly for her manicure treatment, who would always pick at the dry skin around her fingernails. This caused a lot of problems which would often lead to an infection. She had slight dementia and picked at her skin through boredom. It was difficult for the nursing staff and me to try and get her to stop despite our efforts. However, giving her a manicure (when she did not have an infection), made some improvement, especially when I used the nail oil mixture.

EMPHYSEMA

Emphysema is a degenerative disease of the lung tissue. It slowly destroys the tiny air sacs in the lungs over many years. The lungs cannot repair this damage. Emphysema is an irreversible disease. The main symptom of emphysema is a feeling of breathlessness that gradually becomes more severe with time. The damage to the lungs occurs for many years before the effects are felt. While it does not result in as many deaths as lung cancer or heart disease, it is a debilitating illness involving the erosion of the lungs. Cigarette smoking is the main cause of emphysema and it tends to be a late effect of long-term smoking (Quit Victoria 2009; see also Cancer Institute NSW in the Resources and Further Reading section).

I have noticed people suffering from this disease have difficulty in breathing, and it is not very pleasant to witness. People who have this disease are in need of a ventilator most of the time, especially when the disease is more severe. They can have difficulty in their mobility and can become very tired and easily exhausted. Their fingernails are stained from the years of smoking and have dark yellow to brown hues, and the face can have a 'yellow' look along with many lines and wrinkles. The skin has a dry and 'leathery' feel on the clients I have treated. Although a cosmetic cream may help the skin to feel hydrated it has no effect in improving the skin to its full potential, especially if the client continues to smoke. Unfortunately I have seen this: even when the client was using an oxygen mask, she needed to go outside the building to have a cigarette, such was her addiction.

CHRONIC BRONCHITIS

Chronic bronchitis is the excess production of mucus in the lungs' air passages in response to constant irritation by tobacco smoke. Tobacco smoke contains irritant gases that impair the cleaning mechanisms of the lungs. In combination, they result in constant coughing, phlegm production and obstruction of the small airways in the lungs (Quit Victoria 2009; see also Cancer Institute NSW in the Resources and Further Reading section).

Chronic bronchitis is most frequently caused by long-term irritation of the bronchial tubes. Besides tobacco smoke, other influences that can cause bronchitis are allergies, exposure to airborne pollutants, such as dust in the air, and chemicals. The elderly and debilitated are prime targets for complications of acute bronchitis because they are more susceptible to secondary infections.

PNEUMONIA

Pneumonia is inflammation of the lungs, usually caused either by bacteria or a virus. Pneumonia can also be caused by inhalation of a foreign substance, sometimes vomit. The lungs become filled with pus, mucus and other fluids and can no longer function effectively. Oxygen is prevented from reaching the cells and blood. There are many types of pneumonia, most of which are caused by bacterial infection. The bacteria and viruses that cause pneumonia are highly contagious and can be passed on in fluid or saliva from the mouth or droplets from the nose of anyone infected (Ehealth 2009).

Many frail older persons can become infected with pneumonia which leaves them very ill and in some cases has fatal consequences.

VISION IMPAIRMENT

Vision impairment affects many people in all age groups, with most ending up having to wear glasses or contact lenses. Many eye problems can also lead to surgery. Vision impairment is a term that describes various impairments relating to sight and the loss of sight. As people age, eye problems such as cataracts, glaucoma, pterygium and age-related macular degeneration are common, especially among frail older people.

Cataracts are cloudy areas that form in the lens of the eye. The lenses are normally clear. Poor vision results because the cloudiness interferes with light entering the eye. The opacities in the lens scatter the light, causing hazy vision, in the same way that a dirty window scatters light (Optometrists Association Australia 2009a).

Glaucoma is a condition in which the nerve cells which transmit information from the eye to the brain become damaged. This prevents visual information from getting from the retina in the eye to the brain. Glaucoma is often associated with a build-up of pressure in the eye. The eye is filled with fluid which is constantly being replaced. If excessive amounts of fluid are produced, or if it cannot drain away properly, the pressure inside the eye can increase. In some forms of glaucoma, the pressure inside the eye can become extremely high, but in other forms the pressure may remain normal (Optometrists Association Australia 2009b).

Pterygium is a triangular-shaped lump of tissue which grows from the conjunctiva on to the cornea. Pterygia often occur in both eyes, usually on the side of the eye closer to the nose. A pterygium is not cancer. People sometimes confuse pterygia with cataracts (Optometrists Association Australia 2009c).

Age-related macular degeneration is damage or breakdown on the macular. The macular is a very small part of the retina, the light-sensitive tissue of the eye, which is responsible for central vision. This is the part of the retina which produces the finest detailed vision (Optometrists Association Australia 2009d).

I have given beauty therapy to clients who suffer from the above. Many people wear glasses and I have also treated a few clients who were blind since their birth. With older frail persons who have a visual impairment, I found it best to avoid the eyes when giving treatment and best not to apply cosmetics. It is important for a therapist to be aware of the client's visual capacity. If the client cannot see at all, make sure she knows what you are going to do and how you will apply her treatment. Explain to her where things are, if you have moved anything in her room. If you walk with a visually impaired client, do not pull her along, but instead walk with her and allow her to hold on to you. In my experience I have found visually impaired clients who reside in a nursing home are familiar with the home surroundings and can easily walk along corridors to and from their room. Walking with a visually impaired client in their familiar surroundings, I found the task to be easy. I had to let her know only if there were trolleys, people or other objects blocking the corridor.

> For 13 years I had visited a client who was blind from birth. She loved having facial treatments. One day she told me she never knew what it was like to wear any makeup and would love to have enjoyed the pleasure other women had, especially when she was in her teens. I told her: 'Well, you are in luck, because

it is never too late, and I have an idea how you may be able to learn to apply a little bit of makeup.' She was delighted. I taught her how to apply her moisture cream and how to apply face powder and lipstick. We did this by a 'counting' method (see 'Makeup tips for older women' in Chapter 5).

If a client wears glasses, make sure they are clean before returning them after treatment. Many frail clients are unable to keep their glasses clean and this can easily be overlooked.

HEARING IMPAIRMENT

There are two types of hearing loss. One happens when the inner ear or auditory nerve is damaged. This type is permanent. The other kind happens when sound waves cannot reach the inner ear. Earwax build-up, fluid or a punctured eardrum can cause it. Untreated, hearing problems can get worse. Possible treatments include:

- hearing aids
- cochlear implants
- special training
- certain medicines and surgery.

Hearing loss can be caused by:

- heredity
- diseases such as ear infections and meningitis
- trauma
- certain medicines
- long-term exposure to loud noises
- ageing.

(National Institute on Deafness and other Communication Disorders and MedlinePlus 2009)

I have found it difficult at times when an older person will not put in her hearing aid. If she has poor eyesight, communication can be more difficult.

If a client could read, I found if I wrote my request in large print on paper, then she could understand what I was trying to tell her. Most of my elderly clients have found that their hearing aids cause too much ringing and buzzing which can be annoying, and because of this they will not put them in. When dealing with a person who has impaired hearing, ask her if she can put in her hearing aid (that is if she is not wearing it) and encourage her to leave it in until the treatment is over. This has proved satisfactory in many cases.

> Never raise your voice to try and make a hearing impaired person hear. This can only make things worse, with the person feeling intimidated and the therapist ending up with a 'sore' throat. Also, it is very unprofessional to shout at a person with impaired hearing.

PART THREE: NUTRITIONAL IMPAIRMENT

As people age and their dietary needs change, they may eat less. When illness, pain or a disability occurs, nutrient deficiency is often a problem, especially with older frail persons if they do not get sufficient vitamin and minerals from their daily food requirements. There are many factors that can relate to a person's inability to achieve proper nutrient intake. Medication can increase risks of poor nutrition status in older people, due to the effects of drugs on absorption, metabolism and drug nutrient interactions. Disability and losses in everyday personal functions required for everyday independent living are caused by diseases which impair the cells and organs by diseases. The most common conditions with nutritional implications in older people are:

- arthritis
- hypertension

- heart disease

- orthopaedic impairments

- chronic sinusitis

- diabetes mellitus

- cataracts

- deafness or hearing loss

- haemorrhoids

- blindness

- arteriosclerosis

- constipation.

Many frail older people suffer some type of dementia, which also affects nutritional status. Low body mass is quite common in demented older persons, resulting from the other illnesses they may be suffering. Depression is also common among older people who reside in aged-care facilities or who live independently in residential care. Older frail persons living alone can suffer from weight loss and poor nutrition because of their inability to shop, prepare food or feed themselves. This may be due to:

- their disability

- possible impairments in taste and smell (taking oral medications)

- underlying illness

- sore gums or ill-fitting dentures

- lack of appetite, and (in some agitated persons), increased energy needs.

(Tay 2009, pp.89–90)

TEETH AND DENTURES

Many frail older persons have lost most of their teeth and have difficulty in chewing. Some have lost all their teeth and wear dentures for both bottom and top plates. Gum shrinkage is common, which can lead to improperly fitting dentures that can cause soreness in the gums, including gum ulcers. In some cases, this can be known as the hidden pain, as there are frail older persons who are unable to communicate and will suffer in silence unbeknown to the carer. Some indications that a frail person may be having problems with her teeth or gums are:

- dribbling

- sucking on fingers

- continued mouth movements as in chewing

- sensitivity to being touched in or around the mouth

- movement of dentures

- swelling of gums

- bad breath (can also be caused by medication or an illness).

Other factors that can also relate to a person's lack of interest in eating are:

- religious beliefs where certain foods are forbidden

- unpalatability of certain foods

- irritation of the digestive system by certain foods

- unappetising food or food that is too cold

- emotional and physical stress

- loss of zest for life

- other factors that may relate to personal beliefs.

(Tay 2009, pp.91–92)

IMPORTANCE OF WATER INTAKE FOR OLDER PERSONS

Water requirements are particularly important among older persons. Thirst mechanisms are weak, body water is low, the ability to concentrate the urine decreases, and many older people are on diuretics, which cause increased loss of water. Another problem that occurs is when some older people limit their fluid intake to avoid trips to the toilet due to their mobility problems.

A dry skin is often a sign of dehydration and poor nutrition, which is very common in frail older people. The feel and look of skin can signal good or poor nutrition. Lack of proper exercise and insufficient water intake can contribute towards dehydration and constipation, leading to many discomforts and illnesses for the person. In my experience, I have found that many older persons prefer their daily intake of coffee, tea or sweet drink rather than to drink fresh water (Tay 2009, pp.93–94).

SOCIAL DINING FOR LOW CARE RESIDENTS

Older residents in low care are able to feed themselves and find their way to the dining room in a nursing home, or they may go out with family or friends to dine. Many enjoy the social aspect of meeting in the dining room and having conversation with the other residents at meal times. 'Social eating' encourages older people to eat regularly, reducing the risks of becoming nutritionally impaired. In some nursing homes the residents are seated at different tables each week so that they can get to know the other residents. Some of my clients have told me that they like this system, while others have said that they do not like 'changing'. A pleasant atmosphere, good company and the decoration of a table setting can induce a healthy appetite for most people. I have been impressed by a few dining room settings in the nursing homes I have visited. I found as I entered the room it was like going into a 'classy' restaurant. The tables were set with tablecloths and table napkins, the residents' place cards, proper cutlery (not plastic), clear wine glasses and water glasses. Flowers were in matching vases, placed in the centre of each table, creating a pleasant atmosphere for the residents. Not all dining rooms are set up like this. Some are very basic with just table mats and minimal cutlery. This may be due to safety factors, especially for residents who have poor memory or dementia.

When a person's health declines and her memory is frayed, her dining habits may change. Familiar routines become very important and this includes at meal times. If a client is out of her routine she can become agitated and restless. I have clients on my appointment list who often worry if they are not on time for their meals or are missing out on the tea trolley for their morning or afternoon tea. When a client becomes concerned about her meals I reassure her that the kitchen staff will keep her meal warm or the person with the tea trolley will come into the salon with her tea or coffee while she is having her treatment. On some occasions, if the client is having a manicure or a face mask, she can still have her tea or coffee. This can be an issue when dealing with diabetic clients as they must have their food and fluid intake when required. When I am treating clients in a nursing home I will try to fit in my diabetic clients first, just after meal times, depending what time of the day I visit.

TIPS FOR THE THERAPIST

For the therapist to become familiar with an illness or a disability, it is not necessary to be an expert, but simply to have an idea of how best to work with such conditions. With regard to medication, it is not necessary for the non-medical therapist to know all about various drugs. Just be aware that certain medications can affect the growth of hair, cause dehydration in the skin and weakening of the nails, as well as bruising. With experience the therapist will become familiar with the side effects from some medications, and will find that people taking the same medication may differ in reactions. Knowing this, the therapist will understand that the skin and fingernails may not fully regain optimal health, although there could be improvement if the client continues with regular treatments.

I have been asked many times by people who show little understanding, 'Why give a person treatment if there is no real improvement?' My response is, as long as the person still wishes to continue having treatment, and can cope, she is entitled to have attention, in the same manner as any other person requiring her beauty or natural therapy treatment. Showing attention to a person will give her the satisfaction of knowing that she can look forward to maintaining her nail and skin care routine, even though she knows the treatment may show only 'satisfactory' results. The specific time not to give a treatment is when the individual cannot continue, due to declining health. Client assessment is essential in situations like this, as sometimes a client may wish to continue with her treatment, when realistically it would not be practical. As I have stated previously, the important focus is: quality and care.

CHAPTER 3

Hygiene Practice

PERSONAL HYGIENE

At all times the therapist must be aware of her hygiene procedures. This includes daily procedures in the salon or clinic, and taking care of her client's hygiene, especially when treating older persons and those in palliative care. Personal hygiene standards for the therapist must also be considered before treating a client.

> Do not take the risk of treating clients who have a cold, flu-like symptoms or an infection. This is a quick way of spreading germs to you and to other clients.

THE CLIENT IN THE SALON OR CLINIC

Make sure that:

- each client has clean towels (caps or gowns if necessary) and clean linen for the treatment table

- the client has a clean place to put her things

- all products used for the client's treatment are clean

- all equipment and utensils (tweezers, scissors, files, etc.) are 'salon' standard cleaned

- dirt is removed from the client's face, hands or feet before treatment

- the client is encouraged to use a hand sanitising lotion.

HYGIENE CARE FOR THE THERAPIST

- Wear clean clothes or a protection garment each day, such as an apron, overclothes or uniform.

- Keep shoes clean as they have a tendency to pick up dirt while on your travels.

- Keep hair tidy, fingernails clean and appearance tidy.

- Make sure hygiene practices are carried out before and after client treatments.

    Over the years I found that wearing disposable aprons was a good alternative when I went on my rounds to the nursing homes. It was also advisable to wipe over shoes, especially when I was visiting clients in their own home, in a hospital or in a nursing home. Shoes are often overlooked when it comes to hygiene. After my daily rounds of visits to various venues, I also found it was necessary to have a shower as soon as I arrived home, because I had sometimes picked up strong odours during the course of my visits!

EQUIPMENT HYGIENE

At the end of the day, all equipment must be cleaned thoroughly and left in a sanitising unit overnight or placed in an airtight container. Each day, instruments needed must be placed separately in a fresh paper bag or a sterile bag ready for the next day's rounds. Carry bags and all cosmetic containers should be wiped over. Brushes should be washed in warm water with pure soap or a mild shampoo and gently squeezed under running water, then reshaped to dry on a clean paper towel. The carry bag is then ready for the next day, including disposable items and clean equipment.

HYGIENE STANDARDS IN THE SALON OR CLINIC

In the salon or clinic, clean up after each client, dispose of rubbish, change linen and sanitise equipment, clean treatment table and any other areas that have been used. Each day wipe the floors, window-ledges and any other areas that need cleaning. Clean the waiting room and change water if there are fresh flowers. All objects handled through the day (e.g. door handles, phone, chairs, lights, etc.) should be wiped over with disinfectant. If this becomes a daily practice, the therapist will never fail in hygiene procedures.

> When I am visiting clients, either in their own home, a nursing home or a hospital, I place my used products into a paper bag which can be disposed of safely into a bin. This makes good hygiene practice.

Hand hygiene

It is essential to follow instructions on hand washing procedures when visiting hospitals, nursing homes and other aged-care facilities. The instructions for hand washing are generally placed over the sink used by medical staff and visitors. In a salon or clinic, the therapist should have instructions placed where other staff can read them, and to follow correct procedure for hand washing. Hand washing is an essential part of the therapist's safety practice. Always ensure that hands are clean and washed before, during and after each client's treatment. Dirt on the hands can spread germs to other parts of the body and to other clients. Always use disposable gloves when cleaning dirt from the client's skin and fingernails. Keep tubes or bottles of antiseptic cleanser for hand washing in case there is none available where you are visiting.

> When visiting homes, I generally carry a bottle of tea-tree cleanser and sanitising lotion which I find adequate for my hand washing as well as getting rid of dirt from under the

fingernails. I have found hand sanitisers practical to use when treating a client during their therapy. Although the sanitisers are recommended, they should be used by therapists in conjunction with hand washing procedures.

The rest room

From time to time, clients will want to use the toilet. It is important to keep this area clean and make sure there is a sink with taps that have hot and cold water for the client to wash their hands. Containers of liquid soap and a sanitising lotion should also be provided along with disposable paper hand towels and towelling cloths. A bin should be placed near the sink for the disposable paper. A separate disposable unit or bin can be placed inside the rest room for sanitary disposables. All bins should be lined with a bag that can be disposed of easily, avoiding contact with any soiled items. Gloves should always be worn for extra protection when removing rubbish from a bin into a disposable unit or into a council rubbish bin. After disposing of rubbish, remove gloves and wash hands.

> Refer to your local council or health department for regulations regarding the procedure for disposing of sanitary items.

Disposable gloves

Disposable gloves are for protection and to help prevent contamination of both the practitioner and client. When visiting a client in a nursing home, hospital or private home, it is advisable for the therapist to use disposable gloves for conducting a client's first assessment and for skin analysis. If the therapist is satisfied that the client has no open sores, cuts and infections, the gloves can be removed. Hand washing procedures must then be carried out before commencement of any treatment. Always glove for 'first time' facial waxing, and each time for manicure and pedicure procedures. Wear gloves throughout the treatment if necessary, especially with frail older clients.

LINEN HYGIENE

Linen should be stored away and not exposed to dust particles that circulate in the atmosphere, as the latter are easily absorbed, especially in towelling material. Once the linen is used, place it into a basket ready for laundering. Oiled linen, such as towels and gowns used in a massage treatment, should be placed separately as they can make other linen rancid and smelly. Oily linen should be washed in very hot water. A laundry service is good to use in maintaining the condition of linen, but it can be expensive long term. If laundry is washed on the premises, make sure all soiled linen is washed separately. Hot water is essential in laundering as the steam can disperse unwanted odours, oils and stubborn dirt particles. Use a strong detergent and rinse thoroughly. Clean linen can still house pathogens, therefore it is not a good idea to take it out of the salon or clinic for use with clients residing in hospitals, nursing homes or private homes. Clients in this category should supply their own linen. There are exceptions, however, for hairdressers because of the nature of their treatments: hair dyes and other chemical products used for hair perming and styling will stain linen, and at times this is unavoidable. Using a client's own linen or the nursing home's linen is not an option in these circumstances.

> 'Oiled' linen is any material used during a treatment where spillage and stains accumulate from base oils, essential oils and other oil-based cosmetics. Disposable linen such as face cloths, towels and massage gowns can be an alternative to using linen.

PACKING THE COSMETIC BAG

Beauty therapists

For the beauty therapist who runs a mobile service to nursing homes, hospitals and private homes a cosmetic bag's contents can include disposable accessories as well as reusable items. The therapist may need to include other implements that are not listed below.

STATIONERY

- receipt and invoice books
- pens
- client cards (report files)
- note paper
- business cards
- price list on treatments
- contracts (if necessary)
- advertising brochures
- a Do Not Disturb sign
- an appointment book

COSMETICS

- moisturisers
- cleansers
- exfoliant creams
- face mask (creams, lotions or clays)
- nail polish (not to include resin or formaldehyde)
- fingernail accessories
- brow tinting colour
- antiseptic cleansers
- organic powder (not talc) or cornflour
- wax strips
- wax cleanser
- essential oils

- hand lotion
- eye colour pencils
- tinted moisturisers
- foundation
- concealers
- eye shadows
- lipsticks
- blush
- face powder

As an alternative, mineral makeup may be a better option to use on frail older persons. Make sure it is 'organic' and does not include harmful ingredients.

Utensils (or instruments)

- tweezers
- nail scissors
- nail files
- nail buffers
- cutting scissors (for material and paper)
- wands or brushes for eye brow tinting
- accessories for applying makeup
- cuticle sticks
- stainless steel bowl

Disposables

- cotton pads
- cotton buds
- cotton balls
- face wipes
- paper towels
- strip wax
- tissues
- disposable gloves
- cuticle sticks
- emery boards
- lip brushes
- eye shadow applicators
- mascara wands (come in handy for combing eyebrows)
- apron
- disposable wipes
- paper bags (for disposing of rubbish)
- cleaning cloth
- tissues
- bowls

Cleaning agents

- sanitising lotion
- tea tree oil

- disposable wipes (for cleaning)
- cleansing lotion

First aid accessories

- sticking plasters
- antiseptic cleanser
- disposable gloves
- tweezers
- scissors

Natural therapists

Therapists may find some of the following items useful to include in their treatment bags:

Useful items

- cleaning agents (see above)
- massage creams and essential oils
- stationery (see above)
- first aid equipment (see above)

Disposables

- cotton pads
- cotton buds
- cotton balls
- face wipes
- wipes
- gloves

- aprons

- tissues

- bath powder (not talc) or cornflour

- essential oils

- cleansing lotion

- massage cream

THE CLIENT'S COSMETIC HYGIENE CARE

With changing trends in cosmetic use, men in the latter years have begun to embrace cosmetic use in their daily hygiene care. The following tips apply to both genders.

Many people of all ages overlook the importance of maintaining hygiene care for their cosmetics. Lids are either left off jars or tubes, or put back incorrectly, leaving the product exposed to pollutants, which can cause bad bacteria to multiply, contaminating the cosmetic so that it is no longer suitable for use. Contaminated products can result in skin problems when a person ignores the signs, and continues to use a contaminated product, all in the cause of 'money saving'. All cosmetics should be used within a limited time once a product has been opened. Stale colour makeup should be disposed of regularly, and not kept long term, as it loses colour and texture, not enhancing the skin as it should do. Dirty accessories also add to poor application of cosmetics, which can spread germs from one area of skin to another. In the nursing homes I visit, I find many clients have difficulty in maintaining hygiene product care. As these are the client's personal items, it is not really the responsibility of the staff to check for cleanliness; however, over the years I have encouraged relatives and volunteers to take on this task on a regular basis, if the resident is happy for them to do so. Many were pleased to take on this task and found they appreciated the information learned on cosmetic hygiene.

Some women had their cosmetics out when I came to visit, and asked if I would see if their makeup was clean. While some women were capable of cleaning and taking care of their cosmetics and cosmetic application, many were not. It is with these clients that I would spend a little extra time.

Hygiene tips the therapist can suggest for the client

- *Moisturisers for men and women.* Spatulas should be used when taking a product from a container (see Figure 3.1). Using fingers is another way to spread pathogens (germs) from one part of the body to another.

- *Compressed powders.* Encourage a client to clean her powder puff and this will help prevent the powder becoming dry and cracked. Dry cracks in powder are caused by accumulation of sweat and other dirt particles from the client's skin. This occurs when 'contaminated' powder puffs are placed back into the containers after application. An alternative is to use a disposable cotton pad.

- *Lipsticks.* I have found with many older women their lipstick tubes were worn down to the last trace of colour, and the container has become very dirty. These old lipsticks have been in the possession of the client for many years and thus she does not like to part with them. Another reason may be that it is her favourite colour and is no longer on the market. When a client does not want to change to a new lipstick or stop using her 'old favourite' I have managed to get her to wipe over the lipstick with a tissue after use and I show her how to keep the container clean. Another problem I encounter is that younger women often share their lipsticks, and contamination can occur through infections from a cold sore or other lip infections. Sharing is not an option when it comes to using cosmetics.

- *Eyebrow pencils and eyeliner pencils.* Advise the client to keep them separate from other makeup and keep the pencil lid on. Pencils should be sharpened after use with a suitable eye pencil sharpener.

- *Nail varnish bottles.* Instruct the client how to keep the varnish bottle clean from the build-up of stale polish that accumulates around the rim of the bottle. This mainly happens when the lid is not replaced properly after use and left exposed to the air and other pollutants.

To overcome hygiene concerns, I generally encourage my clients to use disposable cotton pads for applying powder, as it saves time trying to clean powder puffs. All cosmetic containers should be cleaned regularly as should lipstick tubes, powder containers, blusher and eye shadow containers. All accessories should be kept clean. Disposable items are useful, as these are beneficial for older clients who are forgetful about cleaning their products.

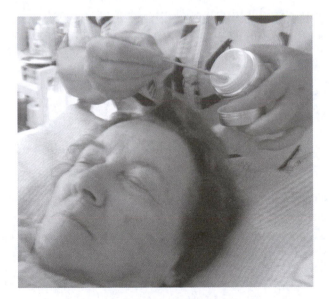

FIGURE 3.1 Use a disposable spatula to take cosmetic cream from a jar to prevent contamination.

PATHOGEN PREVENTION PROCEDURES

Sterilisation

Sterilisation is the killing or removal of all micro-organisms in a material or on an object. Sterility means that there are no living organisms in or on a material when sterilisation is properly carried out. The sterilisation process ensures that even highly resistant bacterial endospores and fungal spores are killed.

Some sterilisation techniques are very dangerous when used in a salon or clinic. It is impractical and impossible to completely sterilise equipment and surfaces in the salon. Sterilisation is mainly required for hospital procedures. Some salons will have a small sterilising unit to store their instruments, however, this can be misleading as some of the old model units are really 'sanitising units'. These ultraviolet (UV) cabinets don't kill bacteria pathogens but inhibit their growth and are ideal for storing implements once they are cleaned. However, the therapist needs to turn the instruments over as the UV only works on one side. Proper sterilisation procedures must be carried out by the therapist if treatments involve any form of skin piercing such as:

- tattooing

- body piercing (including ear piercing)

- cutting of cuticles and skin wicks

- removal of dead skin and blackhead extraction and other activities that include skin penetration.

Failure to sterilise contaminated equipment between clients has the potential to transmit infectious diseases.

There are some basic home methods that a therapist can use to sterilise instruments.

- *Baking.* Place instruments on a clean oven tray, put into an oven at 350°F, or 150°C for 45 minutes.

- *Boiling.* Allow the water to come to boiling point, immerse instruments into water and boil for 20 minutes.

- *Autoclave.* Steam instruments at 250°F, 125°C, for 30 minutes.

A pressure cooker is another method of sterilising instruments, as it is as good as autoclaving. It steams to 130°C degree heat and can kill almost anything.

Instruments can be bagged separately and sealed until further use, or placed in a sterilising or sanitising unit.

> When I visit clients who reside in a nursing home or in their own home, I use a sterile paper bag for each client (name written on the front of the bag) then I place the accessories and other items inside the bag. Reusable items are placed separately in another small bag. This is a safe way to prevent cross-infection from using the same implement for another client.

Disinfection

Disinfection is reducing the number of pathogenic micro-organisms to the point where they pose no danger of disease. Disinfection is the second level of decontamination and a higher level than sanitation. Disinfection is almost as effective in the salon as sterilisation, except that most disinfectants do not kill spores.

Disinfectants are not safe to use on skin and can cause irritation and skin damage. Disinfectants can be potentially dangerous if used incorrectly, therefore it is always wise to read the manufacturer's instructions before use. The supplier should always provide a label with safety instructions for the correct procedure of using disinfectants. High quality disinfectants must perform a variety of special jobs in the salon or clinic. They must be able to destroy:

- harmful bacteria

- pathogenic viruses

- fungi.

A hospital level disinfectant must perform all of these functions and would be suitable for use in salons and clinics.

Method of disinfecting instruments

Clean instruments first and get rid of any residue (dirty instruments will contaminate the disinfectant). Place the washed instruments in a glass container filled with a disinfectant solution for approximately 20 minutes, depending on the instructions on the label. Place a lid over the container. Cloudy disinfectant must be changed immediately. Change the solution according to the manufacturer's instructions. Do not leave the instruments in too long as some disinfectants can cause corrosion and they will be unusable subsequently.

> I recommend the use of stainless steel utensils or instruments that don't corrode in strong disinfectants.

Sanitisation

The lowest level of decontamination is called sanitation or sanitising. Sanitising reduces bacterial numbers on implements and equipment. Sanitisation may simply refer to thorough washing with only soap or detergent. A low level of pathogens can be considered safe, so sanitisation is a very effective form of decontamination.

Sanitising units

These units are used to store instruments that have been immersed in a disinfectant. Once the instruments have been cleaned they are placed in the unit where they remain free from contamination. However, they do not protect against viruses and all bacteria, therefore proper sanitising procedures are essential.

Other forms of sanitising are:

- using detergent and water
- antiseptics for skin and cuts

- hand washing

- soaking utensils in a solution.

Sanitisation is a vital part of maintaining a professional establishment.

INFECTIONS AND IMMUNITY

Bacteria

Bacteria are so small they can only be seen through a microscope. Although there are many thousands of species and strains known they tend all to look much the same. Bacteria are the most plentiful organisms on earth and they can multiply at an incredible speed. Bacteria are found in all living organisms and decaying matter. Most bacteria are harmless; others can cause problems. The problem-causing bacteria are pathogenic, that is disease-causing, and are the most common causes of infection and disease in humans. Bacteria will invade any living plant or animal tissue and feed on living matter. They breed rapidly and spread disease by producing toxins (poisons) in the tissue they invade.

Viruses

Viruses are infectious agents too small to be seen with a light microscope. They are not cells. When viruses invade cells, they display some properties of living organisms and so are on the borderline between living and non-living. They enter a healthy cell, grow to maturity and reproduce, often destroying the cell. Viral warts, hepatitis, chicken pox, influenza, measles, mumps and the common cold are all examples of viral infections that can be transferred through casual contact with an infected person.

> The therapist should never visit a frail person in her home or residing in a nursing home while she has a cold or any viral infection, as frail older people and infirm people are very vulnerable to infection.

Fungi

Fungi are plant-like parasites and include all types of fungi and mould. Both are contagious but only fungi are a threat and can affect the nails (in the hands and feet) and other areas of the body. Certain types of fungi may appear white or discoloured, especially under the fingernails and toenails. They can spread towards the cuticle. As the condition matures, the discoloration becomes darker. Clients with a fingernail or toenail infection must be seen by their medical practitioner or podiatrist. Fungi infection found in a nursing home resident must be reported to the RN by the therapist, as fungal infections are very common and contagious among the frail and elderly. Fungal and bacteria infections can be avoided by proper sanitary precautions.

IMMUNITY TO INFECTION

All living organisms have defences against infection. Immunity is the body's ability to recognise and dispose of substances which it interprets as foreign and harmful to its well-being. Immunity against disease is a sign of good health, and can be natural, naturally acquired or artificially acquired.

- *Natural immunity.* A healthy body is able to fight off harmful foreign bodies before they grow and cause disease. Our body is capable of fighting infections in three ways:

    1. by a protective layer of unbroken skin

    2. by natural secretions of perspiration and digestive juices

    3. by white blood cells that kill pathogens.

- *Naturally acquired immunity.* This occurs when antibodies fight off a disease and remain in the blood, ready to fight another attack should the disease return.

- *Artificially acquired immunity.* An injection of serum or vaccine is administered into the body which introduces a small dose of dead or disabled pathogens. The introduced substance fools the immune system into making antibodies that can fight that particular disease.

IMMUNISATION CONCERNS FOR THE THERAPIST

The therapist may want to consider vaccination, especially where body contact with another person is part of their daily services. The therapist who deals with skin piercing or skin penetration procedures would be at a higher risk if they do not keep their vaccinations up to date or practise proper hygiene care. This should apply to all therapists whether they are working in a salon or clinic or from their home as a sole operator. It is best for the therapist to discuss this matter with her doctor or health-care practitioner.

A vaccination against influenza is an annual injection designed to protect an individual from most current viral strains. It has been recommended by health authorities for people working in the health-care industry and for people with chronic conditions to consider updating their vaccinations. Older people and debilitated persons are also very vulnerable to infections. Should the therapist be suffering from any flu-like symptoms, or from a cold, it is advisable she does not treat a client as such illnesses can be contagious.

For more information on vaccinations, refer to workplace safety practices or your local health department. (See the Resources and Further Reading section at the back of this book.)

CHAPTER 4

Fingernail and Skin Care Tips

COMMON FINGERNAIL PROBLEMS

Older frail people probably only require a basic manicure. It is not necessary or profitable to expand beyond the limit of what a person can cope with. Some women like to have colour on their nails, while many just prefer a clear varnish or none at all. No matter how qualified or experienced a therapist may be, it is not necessary or advisable to give a pedicure treatment to people who are in high care. This is because of the many underlying conditions that can occur in frail people, such as poor circulation, infections and other internal factors. Toenail and feet treatments are always referred on to a podiatrist or a medical doctor. Extra care must be given for diabetics in manicure procedures due to their poor circulation and poor healing capacity. Reflexologists must also be aware of these problems when giving treatment.

The most common nail problems related to frail older people are:

- thickening with age
- external damage
- brittleness
- peeling
- furrowing
- excessive growth
- splitting

- cuticle skin growing up the nail

- hang nails

- discolouration

- loss of nail

- fungal infections

- ingrown nail

- thin nails

- flaky nails (shedding of top layer of nail plate)

- loss of a nail or nails

- deformed nails

- bacterial infections.

The main causes of most problems may relate to:

- illness

- medication

- damage to nail

- poor circulation

- hygiene neglect

- improper manicure and pedicure procedures

- chemicals

- nail polish removers and coloured nail varnish

- poor nutrition

- dirt or excrement left under nails which causes weakness and infections

- or, simply, ageing.

The constant use of hands without hygiene attention is also a major problem for fingernails in poor condition. Cuticle care is so important in the frail elderly. A common problem is when the cuticle skin attaches to the nail plate and starts to grow up towards the free-edge of the fingernail when left untreated. (This may be caused by some internal disorder.) At this stage the fingers become very tender and sore and it is very difficult to push the cuticle skin back. Nail oils (essential and base oils used for fingernail and toenail treatment) or cuticle cream will help soften the cuticles, and with time and patience, after many treatments, there can be a slight improvement for some clients.

> I have seen the condition of cuticle skin growing up the nail at its worst on a woman where the nails are hardly visible and the skin had thickened. (This possibly may have been the result of long-term arthritis she had suffered in her fingers and hands.) Massaging the hands with essential oils gave comfort to this woman. Unfortunately as her condition deteriorated she could not cope with any further treatment due to her frailty and sensitivity.

Bacterial infections

Bacterial infections can easily spread if fingernail care is neglected. Signs of an infection are redness and swelling and pain around the fingernail skin folds, which become very sore and painful for the client. The infection can turn septic causing pus to accumulate in the affected area. Common causes are poor hygiene, improper manicure or pedicure procedures, frequent exposure to water and untreated wounds. *Paronychia* is when the cuticle becomes detached, causing the nail to loosen and fall off. *Onychia* is when the infection has spread to the matrix and nail bed. Bacterial infections occur frequently in the fingernails of the frail elderly, mainly due to poor hygiene and poor manicure procedures.

> This is one of the reasons I would like to see more trained people working on the frail to help prevent such problems occurring.

COLOURED NAILS – WHAT DO THEY MEAN?

The nail plate can vary in colour and many conditions may be the result of poor circulation, a fungus or bacterial infection, an illness, vitamin deficiency or from topical or oral medications, an injury or the use of coloured nail polish.

Internal problems with coloured nails

To most people the word 'coloured nails' generally refers to the use of coloured nail varnish. To the health-care practitioner and beauty therapist it can have a different meaning. Treating the fingernails of a frail older person can be different from treating the fingernails of a person in a salon. This is because there are many underlying problems a person may have, and the nails are the windows that can relate to internal disorders, showing a multitude of hues according to what the person may be suffering from. Fingernails can be the first clue to serious illness. Not all clients who may be suffering from some of the symptoms listed below will show colour in their nails.

White to pink shades

I have noticed on some older women who are taking blood thinning medication, their nails can be brittle and the colour hue may either show very white or white with pink near the cuticles, or on top along the line of the free-edge. In some cases the pink can spread down from the free-edge to the middle of the nail. If the client has heart problems there may be a definite show of pink streaks across the top of the nail and on some other areas there can also be a slight tinge of blue at the base of the nail. The free-edge of the nail may be white or brittle. Diabetics may also show these signs.

Blue nails

This is mainly an external problem caused through an injury. Internally it may relate to poor circulation, emphysema or lung disease. Diabetics may also show these signs.

Yellow nails

When the nails look streaky (due to the prominent long horizontal ridges) and the base of the nail appears thick, flaky and coming away from the nail bed, this may relate to a defective lymphatic drainage. It could also be the result of a fungal infection. Another problem that may relate to yellow nails is *jaundice* in the nail. The nail may show a pale yellow hue and the nail itself will appear weak and will easily split at the free-edge. Some diabetics may also show these symptoms.

Purple nails

May be related to poor oxygen intake or circulation problems.

Red nails

Redness in the nail or around the nail and finger may indicate the beginning of an infection. A reddish brown hue may also relate to folic acid deficiency. Other possibilities may be due to heart disease, high blood pressure or a stroke.

Green nails

This shows that the nail has an infection and should be treated by a medical practitioner or podiatrist. Do not work around a nail that shows an infection. It may also be caused by an allergy to cleaning agents or emphysema.

Dark brown to black

Should any pigmented longitudinal streaks appear in a nail it may indicate a melanoma and the client should be seen by a medical practitioner. Do not treat the nail if the nail shows any of these signs. Brown spots under the nails may indicate psoriasis or a deficiency of folic acid or protein or vitamin C. Black nails may indicate signs of anaemia, a deficiency in vitamin B12, bacterial infection, chronic kidney disease, liver disease and other internal disorders.

Nail varnish

> The colour showing in the nail will come from the nail bed if it is an internal disorder. An external injury or the over-use of nail colour varnish will show up on the nail plate.

Continuing to use nail colour on frail women can cause the nails to become weak and very discoloured, leaving a yellowish to brown hue. It is best not to paint colour on the nails if this problem occurs. Sometimes this can be a difficult task, especially if the client insists on having a colour applied on the nails. To overcome this problem I have frequently asked a relative or carer to remove the polish after a few days to allow the nails 'breathing space' before the client's next appointment. Unfortunately some relatives and carers will continue to paint the frail person's nails, which can make the situation much worse. An application of fresh polish painted over the old polish will cause a build-up of polish, with the old stale nail polish causing the nails to weaken further. This also causes the nails to split along the free-edge and fray.

> These problems keep occurring mainly because well-intentioned relatives, friends and volunteers try to give the woman a quick manicure or pedicure using utensils that have not been cleaned properly. This is the quickest way for frail people to pick up infections which may cause other disorders in the nails. Relatives will try and save money by not having professional help from a

beauty therapist. Unfortunately, in the long run, the frail person receiving treatment is worse off from the good intentions and false economy. Once the condition worsens, it is difficult to maintain reasonably healthy looking nails for the person, especially if the relatives or visitors continue to use the same procedures.

TREATING HANDS AND FINGERNAILS

Over the years I have found it is best to maintain a basic manicure procedure when treating frail persons. It is not necessary to introduce 'fancy' nail art or new fashion trends. Older frail women would prefer to have their nails kept short and maintained.

In my experience, very few older women like to use coloured nail polish, although some women will ask for a clear polish.

Should a person show any abnormal colour in the fingernails or toenails, do not apply any nail varnish. It may indicate an internal imbalance. Clear nails are essential for diagnostic purposes. Do not use any nail varnish, clear or coloured in this situation, especially if the client is going to have surgery or any other medical treatment.

NAIL POLISH AND NAIL POLISH REMOVER

If the client wants to have coloured varnish applied to her fingernails, I have found it is best to stay with light colours as they are not as harsh on the nails as the dark-coloured varnishes and also do not stain as much. There are new brands of colour polish on the market at present that do not include formaldehyde and toluene, which have been known to cause an allergy to some women. These new colours may be a better option to use on older persons. When removing varnish from the nails, use a non-acetone polish remover as these are less likely to cause an allergic reaction. However, the constituents in a polish remover can affect sensitive people, and they may cause symptoms such as sneezing, coughing, difficulty in breathing, itching, a rash and watery eyes.

If a client should show any of these symptoms do not use any nail colour or nail polish remover.

SIMPLE TIPS

- Use disposables where possible.

- Use gloves when necessary.

- Keep hands clean and sanitised.

- Do not push cuticles back if the client can feel pain or the skin may tear.

- Use creams or essential nail oils to remove dead skin around the cuticles and to remove stubborn dirt.

- Use props where necessary.

- Cut across the nail when shortening the fingernail; do not cut nails too short.

- Use a disposable nail file when filing nails.

- Use a light colour nail varnish without too many harmful ingredients.

- Use antiseptic cleansers or nail oils for cleaning nails.

   A trained therapist could be the link in education on maintenance in nail care for volunteers and relatives of nursing home residents and people in care. Between the client's appointments, the carers could assist in the client's daily care, which would help eliminate some of these problems.

SKIN CARE TIPS

As the ageing process continues into the 60s and beyond, certain changes in the skin are more visible. The skin becomes dehydrated and thinner. It is vulnerable to the external environment, which can contribute to many skin problems. Loss of elastic fibres in the dermis and decreasing resilience will cause the skin to become loose and wrinkled. Many spots, skin growths and marks appear on some individuals. The cells in the tissues regenerate more slowly and cell repair slows and poor circulation also causes slower healing and skin repair. It is not only older persons who will have wrinkles or skin complaints, as these may be due to genetic makeup and an earlier active healthy lifestyle (Tay 2009, pp.103–104).

Older persons can suffer with a multitude of skin disorders and minor skin complaints. The therapist may be familiar with many of them but may not know how to address them when it comes to treating frail older people. Treating an older person's skin is similar to treating a client in the salon or clinic, but the difference is that some older persons in care are under medical supervision and are being treated with medical creams and oral medication for their skin disorders. When a person is under medical care, this takes precedence over any non-medical treatments. This is where the therapist cannot expect to heal or treat a skin condition achieving the same results as are possible for a client in a salon or clinic. However, satisfactory results can occur when regular treatments are applied, such as giving a 'light' facial using a minimal amount of cosmetics or using the client's creams best suited for her skin. In my experience, I have found that many clients with skin disorders are content to have a light facial or a face reflexology treatment and often feel good afterwards, even though they know that their skin problem may not completely heal. In cases where the client is on a topical medicated cream, or taking oral medications for their skin condition, I apply a limited amount of cosmetics, or essential oils, just enough not to irritate the skin or dislodge any scabs or sores. An assessment will enable the therapist to judge what is best for the client.

COMMON SKIN DISORDERS IN OLDER PERSONS

There are a few positive results with frail clients when they have a regular facial or face reflexology, as both can help improve the texture of the skin and leave the skin looking clean and the client feeling refreshed. If a person is not using any medical creams or taking oral medications the results for skin care treatment can be more effective.

Most minor skin problems can be dealt with in much the same way as for a client in a salon, except the treatments may differ and the therapist may find themselves in a position where they are unable to 'remedy' them. Severe skin problems are treated by a medical practitioner, not by a non-medical practitioner.

These are common skin ailments that can occur on frail and older persons, followed by a few simple tips in how to deal with some of them:

- actinic lentigo (liver spots)

- dermatitis (eczema, allergies and rashes)

- telangiectatic angiomas (broken capillaries and spider veins)

- vitiligo (white and pink patches)

- scars and cysts

- milia (whiteheads)

- rosacea (red flushing)

- discoid lupus

- circulation and vascular disorders

- bruising

- actinic keratosis

- skin cancers

- seborrhoeic keratosis (large raised lumps or warts)

- angiomas (red spots)

- fibroepithelial polyps (skin tags)

- pustules and papules (pimples and blind pimples)

- comedones (blackheads)

- dehydration and skin thinning

- warts

- psoriasis

- burns.

Dehydration and skin thinning

Frail older people have thinner, fragile skins due to the conditions previously mentioned. A fragile skin can tear easily if implements nick or cut the skin or when pressure is too heavy. Once the skin breaks or tears it is vulnerable to infections. If the client is on blood-thinning medication, a wound can take longer to heal. Caution with waxing and massage procedures should be considered when dealing with fragile skin. The skin must be firm, but not pulled too tightly during a waxing procedure, otherwise it can tear easily and cause bruising and damage. This is why it is important for the therapist to use light pressure on fragile skin with any therapy treatments. Dehydration is another factor in causing the skin barrier to break down. Spots and marks like whiteheads can appear and they become hard and difficult to disperse. Many older people do not have the opportunity to have regular facial treatments and whiteheads can result from the build-up of dead skin cells and dry skin that can cause the sebum under the skin to become trapped. I have found when a client has regular facials, especially with face reflexology, some of the whiteheads shrink or disperse on their own. Never try to squeeze them out or pierce them, as this can lead to an infection in frail skins. Applying moisturising creams, hydrating gels and a base oil can help to hydrate a dry skin. It doesn't take much to see improvement to the skin when it responds to the application of cream or oil.

Bruising

Bruising is common in frail and sensitive skin. Causes can arise from injections, catheters, bumping, falling and the force of heavy pressure. Other causes are from poor circulation and some medication. When a catheter is inserted into the body, bruising can occur and spread around the affected area. Do not treat around the area where there is a catheter. This also applies to an area that has been recently pierced with a needle.

Frail clients who have some mobility can be unsteady on their feet and are prone to falls. Besides bruising, a fall can lead to many other problems such as fractures and infections if the skin should break. The skin can appear bruised especially in the arms, face and legs, but this could be due to vascular and circulation problems. Poor circulation is common in the legs and diabetics can be prone to this condition. It can look worse when oedema (swelling) occurs and it can be very painful for the client. Do not treat the legs or feet when a client has this condition. The feet and the toenails can also be affected. The client can lose her toenails through poor circulation and can easily become affected with psoriasis and infected with fungi. Decaying tissue is not pleasant to experience as the odour can be very strong and sickly. Bruising in the arms and hands can be by injections, catheters, a fall or bump or by other injuries. The face can appear to have a 'bruised' look with different colour hues that are more likely to be related to broken capillaries, a skin disorder or immune disorder or from hormonal changes.

Broken capillaries

Broken capillaries are more common when the skin thins and some older persons can have more problems with broken capillaries than others. Broken capillaries are a network of small arterioles and venules that branch out like spider's legs and they are visible close to the surface of the skin. This can be disfiguring to some clients. A little colour makeup applied to the face and neck may help minimise some of the redness, but it won't completely hide the veins unless a heavier application is applied, which may be okay for younger persons but is not really advisable for frail older clients. Use light pressure when treating delicate areas.

Rosacea

Rosacea is another disorder that causes the face to go red and the capillaries to stand out. In some cases cysts and papules can occur if the condition is severe. Severe rosacea needs to be treated by a medical practitioner. The pink colour which forms is due to the increased blood flow created as a result of the infection. Many older people can suffer from this condition and it is best not to put too much pressure on the face when giving treatments. Mild rosacea can be treated with beauty therapy, face reflexology and aromatherapy. Light pressure is required when giving a treatment.

Discoid lupus

Discoid lupus is characterised by a rash that appears on the face, neck and scalp, and it does not affect internal organs. This rash is over the cheeks and bridge of the nose, in the shape of a butterfly. It can range in colour from dark red to even purplish or just pink, it can be 'blotchy' or solid, and is usually not raised. The rash can be mildly scaly. It does not itch. It can come and go, lasting hours, days, weeks or longer. It can either worsen over time or fade. Lupus can sometimes be confused with rosacea as both have similar rash patterns on the face with the 'butterfly' look over the nose, cheeks and chin. This condition needs medical attention and most sufferers can be sensitive to cosmetics. Do not treat a client when they have a 'flare-up' of lupus as they may be experiencing burning and pain.

Dermatitis hepeitformis (the gluten rash)

This rash is similar to discoid lupus and tends to spread all over the body, leaving the person with intense itching and a burning sensation. Clusters of small blisters persistently break out on the elbows, knees, buttocks, back or scalp. These symptoms are the hallmarks of dermatitis hepeitformis (DH), a skin manifestation of coeliac disease. DH affects many people with coeliac disease, and those who are gluten intolerant.

> In 2010 I suffered with this skin rash for months and it took a long time before I was actually diagnosed with dermatitis hepeitformis. I was given certain creams to rub over the rash, all to no avail. It was later I realised that this rash is connected to gluten and with the help of my dermatologist I was put on a gluten-free diet along with a lactose-free diet and found that the rash finally disappeared after three months of agony with itching and burns, which did not help with my other health issues. I was not very familiar with coeliac disease gluten intolerance and soon found myself changing over to a new lifestyle and diet after diagnoses. Unfortunately more and more people are being diagnosed as coeliac or gluten intolerant each day, and there are many who have the disease and are not aware of it. The therapist must be very careful when using any product on the skin of a person with coeliac disease or someone suffering gluten intolerance. Vegetable and nut oils may not be an option. Cosmetics should be carefully checked to ensure they do not contain derivatives from nuts, seeds or gluten products.

Varicose veins

This condition is very common in many older persons. Be careful when working on those with varicose veins. If they are large and lumpy avoid treating those areas.

Varicose ulcers

These ulcers are due to the skin breakdown following blood stasis or stagnation (poor circulation). It can start with redness (erythema), itchiness, dryness and skin breakdown leading to ulcers. The appearance on the legs can show various hues ranging from pink to purple and blue and, on some clients, scaling of dead skin cells.

Ulcers

Skin ulcers are a common occurrence among frail persons, especially those who have poor mobility with circulation issues and broken skin. Another concern with ulcers is bed sores (decubitus ulcers). These can occur when a client is kept in bed and pressure on the skin can cause the skin to tear and an infection to occur, thus creating sores. Rubbing against bed linen and crossing of ankles can add pressure if the person stays in one position for a long time. It is important that a client is turned regularly in her bed to prevent pressure to the body. Bony prominences such as the knees, elbows, hips, ankles and heels are areas that can easily be affected. Ulcers can eventuate from any inflammatory area, especially among the frail. Do not treat any area that looks inflamed.

Skin marks and skin spots

- *Brown spots (actinic lentigo).* The skin can have numerous combinations of skin marks and spots. They appear on the skin as a person ages. Some brown spots are similar to freckles but are larger and can range in colour from a light brown to dark brown, to black, depending on a person's skin tone. Mostly, they are found on areas that have been exposed to the sun.

- *White or pink spots and patches (vitiligo).* The pigment-producing cells have been damaged either by an injury, illness, burns or a hormonal disorder. Other causes could be genetic. The most common areas I have noticed are the arms, legs and face. Some makeup camouflage may be helpful for the face and hands.

- *Cherry angiomas* or cherry moles are harmless little red spots or blotches that can appear anywhere on the body. They range in colour from a light pink to a cherry red (hence the name). In some people they can be dark purple.

- *Skin tags* (medical name, acrochordon) are harmless fibroepithelial polyps that grow in areas under the armpits, under and along the bust line, around the neck and on the eyelids. They can also appear on other parts of the body. They have a tendency to grow more on older women and overweight women. Clothes and jewellery rubbing over the skin tags will stimulate blood flow and this encourages them to grow larger.

It is alright for older persons with skin marks and skin spots to have beauty therapy and other body therapies, providing that the marks or spots are not infected, or show any changes in their size or colour for freckles, warts or moles.

Actinic keratosis

These rough red scaly patches appear like warts and occur on the face, neck, hands and forearms as a result of sun exposure in early life. The sores form a crust; the crust falls off and then reforms. They do not heal normally and if left untreated they may have a tendency to become cancerous. From these rough patches a cutaneous horn can grow and resemble hard dry scaly lumps or long horn. They are not painful, more of a nuisance for the client. They can become infected if the client picks at them and causes them to bleed. The client can have treatment but the therapist must be careful not to remove a scab or work near the area that is affected.

Seborrheic dermatitis

This condition affects the scalp and face. It is a chronic condition that can range from a mild to a severe form of dermatitis. It can happen at any age, but becomes worse in older age and affects men more frequently than women. It causes redness, flaking and irritation on many parts of the body especially in parts of hair growth on the head, the scalp and eyebrows. The eyebrows can be affected and can have clumps of yellowish plaque along the eyebrow line and between the brows near the bridge of the nose. I have seen yellow clumps of plaque along the nose and between the two nose grooves. (This can also be due to lack of hygiene care.) The skin can appear shiny, red and inflamed, becoming infected and damaged. This condition can be caused through cosmetics, colour dyes and sun exposure. In mild cases, the therapist can treat the client, but creams suitable for hypersensitive skins should be used. Calendula, almond and avocado oils may help to soothe inflammation. Severe cases should be treated by medical practitioners.

Seborrheic warts (seborrheic keratosis)

These warts are rough and can resemble moles. They are harmless growths that are slightly raised and feel rough and dry. They can range from small to large, and range in colour from a light brown to a dark brown and black on olive or darker skins. They are harmless growths but are annoying when clothing rubs over the surface of the wart. They mostly grow on the sides of the forehead, along the hair line or sides of the face, under the bust line and on the backs of the hands. They can be removed but have a tendency to grow back. I have found it is okay to treat clients with warts as long as I did not work near the wart. They can be covered with makeup for disguising on a younger person.

> I have found that some older women can have large warts and long strands of thin dark or coarse hair that will grow down and around the warts. This mainly happens along the sides of the face. The area of the skin can be very dry and scaly although the

warts can have an 'oily' feel. It is better to tweeze the unwanted hair away from the wart than trying to wax over them. Facial cleansing and light exfoliation is okay, providing pressure is not too heavy.

Moles

In older persons, the most common moles I have found are the flat translucent ones that grow on the face with hair protruding. They can also grow along the eyebrow line and can cause the eyebrows to become wiry, coarse or to grow unevenly. Most are translucent. Other moles can be found on any part of the body and they are either translucent or pink and are slightly raised. Darker moles on older persons may need to be regularly checked by their doctor. Darker moles can have a tendency to change.

> Some flat translucent moles can accumulate around the chin of middle-aged women and the hairs can be very coarse. In some instances, they can be difficult to remove by waxing, therefore careful tweezing is best. If the hairs are too strong to remove, it is better to leave the hair until it grows longer. Aggravation of hair removal can cause the hair in the mole to become more inflamed and it may later develop cysts and scarring.

> Darker moles are more noticeable on people with olive skin and those with darker complexions.

Skin cancers

Some older people can have skin cancers, more commonly the basal cell carcinomas that appear as bumps and are slow growing. They may appear translucent, but if left untreated they can turn into raised pearly borders. They can develop into ulcers and affect the eye area and around the nose.

Squamous cell carcinoma has a high rate of cure if treated at an early stage. It grows quickly and turns into an ulcerated lump that does not heal. The areas that are affected are the neck, face and back of the hands. Many of my older clients have had skin cancers removed more than once as some cancers had a tendency to reappear. I find it best not to treat a client until the wound has healed. When the client has finished using her topical medicated creams, I may introduce cosmetics and oil treatments into her beauty therapy and face reflexology treatments which had proved satisfactory. If the cancer was treated early before developing into a large lump, I found it possible for me to treat a client not long after the cancer was removed. However, it is best to keep away from the area that had been affected until it is completely healed.

SAFETY TIPS FOR THE THERAPIST

1. Assess the client before treatment.

2. Do not treat a client if they are being treated by a doctor for a severe skin disorder.

3.   Do not use heavy pressure on frail older people.

4. If you do not know what the skin problem is, ask the client or medical staff before giving treatment.

5. Do not treat a client if you think it is not safe to do so.

6. Do not use pore strips, they may cause a fragile skin to tear.

7. Do not attempt any skin piercing on frail older people.

8. Report to the medical staff if the client's skin marks or moles have changed.

9. Document the entire client information in their report file after each treatment.

10. Focus on the quality and care given to the client.

CHAPTER 5

Cosmetics and Beauty Therapy

UNDERSTANDING THE USE OF COSMETICS

There are many brands of cosmetics on the market today, many claiming to be pure and natural, or better than most other brands. As beauty therapists we need the correct tools to work with, and this includes the right cosmetic that is going to enhance our business and the best products for our clients' needs. We may be led into believing that the product we work with is the best on the market and it will bring everlasting results, as the manufacturer tells us, with a rewarding bonus from the sales we make. In reality all this 'jargon' will go well in the average beauty salon and the customer is happy to comply with the beauty therapist's advice on the quantity she should buy to be able to maintain a healthy skin. For work with frail and infirm persons, it can be a completely different matter. The cosmetic brand the therapist is using in the salon may not be suitable for such persons. In many cosmetics, there are ingredients that can be harmful. Harmful ingredients can cause added problems to a client's skin, especially if she has skin problems related to illness or medication. The best option is not to use any cosmetic listed with a lot of harmful ingredients. This is where it is handy to have a textbook or search the internet regarding ingredients in cosmetics. Most contemporary cosmetics list their ingredients externally on jars and tubes. In my view I would avoid any cosmetic that does not comply with these rules, as ignorance of what is in a product can be a risk, especially if the client should have an allergic reaction. However, there are many products on the market today that offer a variety of natural harmless ingredients which may be suitable for clients with delicate skins.

Cosmetic ingredients

Understanding cosmetic ingredients is a complex subject. You would probably need to have a science or chemistry degree to fully comprehend how substances interact with each other and with living cells. Today the beauty industry and natural therapy industry are big business and most training schools can offer postgraduate courses in studying the chemistry of 'cosmetic ingredients' and herbal plants for the student to gain their qualifications in a certificate or a diploma degree. This enables the therapist to have a good background knowledge of their product and to be able to advise clients on the best application of skin care for their everyday needs. Postgraduate education is essential in business building. It enables the therapist to maintain and grow their business in the ever-changing economic world.

In my experience, an understanding of cosmetic ingredients can be gained by reference to cosmetic textbooks covering this topic. I have found that research through the internet displays multiple connections to various sites and huge amounts of information. The therapist then has the advantage of keeping up to date on the latest research on cosmetic and herbal ingredients. The most important information the therapist needs to know is where the ingredients originate from, and what are their functions: are they toxic or non-toxic, and what are their side effects? Harmful ingredients are known to cause a range of severe reactions in some people such as allergies, stinging, rashes, hives, burning, dryness and swelling. Frail elderly persons are vulnerable to harsh products as most have thin skin and a high sensitivity. Nail varnish can cause facial dermatitis in some people because of sensitivity to the ingredients that are in some nail colours, such as toluene sulphonamide-formaldehyde resin. Strong fumes from varnish can also cause a client to cough, sneeze or itch. If such responses occur, do not use any nail varnish in a manicure.

Remember, old nail varnish and its continued use will also add problems to the skin as well as the fingernails and toenails.

THE USE OF SORBOLENE CREAMS

Sorbolene is one of the most used cleansers and moisturisers for dehydrated and sensitive skin and widely used by many older persons. Sorbolene creams are made up by most cosmetic companies, each adding 'varying' ingredients. Although some of these brands may be appropriate to use on some people, they may not be suitable for others. Some sorbolene creams can cause sensitivity and skin allergies. In some cases, a few natural ingredients, such as essential oils in minor proportions, mixed in with a basic sorbolene cream, can have a positive effect on the skin of a person with sensitive and dry skin. Combined with these natural ingredients the cream moistens and softens the skin much to the client's satisfaction with no harmful effects.

Clients who have had skin cancer lesions or sores removed can use a night cream or their own cosmetic cream during beauty-care treatment. Always check with the RN or nursing staff first before using any cosmetic on clients with skin cancer disorders (pre- or post-operative).

> Base oils that contain traces of peanuts or other nuts may not be suitable for the frail elderly or those who have an allergy to nuts, either taken orally or applied externally. Almond oil (although from the kernel of a nut) has a milder effect on the skin, and most women I have treated have coped with the oil without having any harsh side effects. Other vegetable and flower oils that have proved effective for eczema and psoriasis sufferers are avocado oil and calendula oil. Calendula oil added to the cream helps sooth inflammation. However, remember no matter how safe a product may claim to be, there will always be a few people who suffer side effects from its use.

APPLICATION OF COSMETIC CREAMS AND LOTIONS

For the best results when applying creams and lotions to the skin of a frail person I have found that a small amount (a drop the size of your thumbnail) is enough for the client's skin to absorb and for the client to feel refreshed, and for her skin to feel smooth and non-greasy. More cream can be added if it is necessary.

> The over-use of moisturisers and body lotions can inhibit the body's natural lipid (oil) production, which is the skin's natural moisturising agent. Lipids are responsible for depositing fatty secretions to the skin, making it smooth.

WHAT COSMETICS SHOULD I USE ON MY CLIENT?

Following a basic understanding of cosmetic and herbal ingredients in skin care, the therapist will need to judge what is the best for their client, and what benefits will they gain from using a certain brand of cosmetics. The therapist may need to ask: Have the cosmetics lived up to the claims when it comes to my clients? Have the cosmetics been satisfactory without causing any harmful reactions?

Using cosmetics that have harmless natural contents is probably best for older people in care. However, always check with the client's skin condition and patch test before applying a new skin-care product. This is why an assessment of a client is important before making a decision on what products are going to be used.

People with severe skin conditions will often use a special cream that has been prescribed by their medical practitioner. In these circumstances the therapist would encourage the client to continue to use the cream after beauty treatment is finished. In some cases a minimum amount of cosmetic or small drop of essential oil may only need to be applied, in conjunction with the client's continued use of her topical skin treatment.

Be aware that some medicated creams that a client is using, may cause drying or irritation, especially to broken skin. Some medications containing preservatives may cause an allergic sensitisation. Another problem is that the client may continue to use her own cosmetic which can aggravate the cause of their condition. Educating some older clients to change their habits, or not to continue to use a favourite cosmetic, is often very difficult as they cannot understand that the cosmetic they have used all their adult life is now causing a skin reaction. If a client is reluctant to change or follow advice, the therapist can only persevere. The most important factor is that it is best not to contribute any further harm to the client's 'frail' skin.

SELLING COSMETICS IN AGED-CARE HOMES

As I mentioned before, not all older persons residing in a nursing home are under full-time care. Some residents are in hostel care (assisted care), which means they are able to come and go from the nursing home as they wish and make their own decisions. Hostel residents are still under a minimum amount of care, therefore it is best to follow the nursing home protocol.

Unit residents are housed in a small self-contained home which is in the complex of the nursing home. The residents in unit housing have complete control of their day-to-day living, and of their expenses. The residents are housed in units because a partner may need more care, or both persons need carer assistance. Many single persons also reside in unit care. The residents are closer to care when required and may have to transfer over to hostel or nursing care when it is time to do so. Visiting a client in a unit is the same as visiting a client in their own home. (See Chapter 8, 'Home Visits and Hospital Visits'.)

Working in a salon, the therapist will meet many older persons who are independent and able to take care of themselves. After a while, a client may find that she can no longer look after herself and thus has to move into a nursing home because of her poor health. The client may request the therapist to visit and continue therapy. The client may also want to continue using familiar cosmetics, and she may want to purchase new products. While the client is still able to be independent in using her cosmetics, this is fine; however, things will change as the client's disability or illness becomes more pronounced and then she may need further attention in care. An illness or disability can prevent a person from attending to her physical needs and this might include cosmetic application. The therapist can decide if they want to continue with a client in care, or recommend the client to another therapist who is more experienced in dealing with frail clients.

At this stage, when a client is in high nursing care, it is not a good idea for the therapist to try and sell them cosmetics because:

- the client's financial circumstances may have changed

- the client is unable to handle her own skin-care routine

- the client receives many gifts of cosmetics for birthdays or Christmas and these are seldom used, and are left on storage shelves where such cosmetics join other toiletries

- staff have no time to attend to the client's skin-care routine each day

- staff will use other creams or the client's medicated cream

- the client is unable to physically apply cosmetics

- confused clients do not understand or remember money transactions or ordering products.

It is best to use common sense. A therapist working with frail older persons will not always find her work profitable. The main consideration is that service and treatments provided by the therapist will make many clients feel happy; a feeling of well-being may result from quality care especially from touch. The experience can be very rewarding for both the therapist and the client.

BEAUTY CARE FOR OLDER PERSONS

The good news is new brands of coloured makeup are currently coming on the market, such as mineral makeup, with some brands claiming to have fewer harmful ingredients and more natural ingredients. These may be beneficial to use on older frail women. On average, the therapist would probably use a minimum amount of coloured makeup on older women. Most women like to be made up with coloured makeup for a special occasion by applying the 'touch' application, or the 'light day' application. It is probably best not to apply colour makeup on women who have severe skin problems. Younger women in care would probably want to have their makeup applied following new trends. However, the tips suggested for older persons can also apply to young women who have delicate and sensitive skin.

> The brand of cosmetic I use for skin care is based on natural ingredients and has proven beneficial for my clients over a period of 18 years. Sometimes I had to use the client's own cosmetic cream or makeup but found at the same time I could still use my cleansing creams which have had no harsh side effects to clients with severe skin conditions. I also incorporated herbal infusions and essential oils into my cosmetic application. I have found that clients who have regular facials over a period of time, have shown some improvement in their skin texture, even though they may continue to use their own cosmetics between their appointments. Regular treatments help improve the skin texture regardless of the client's age.

FACIALS

Preparing a client for treatment

The methods for treating older people with facials, face reflexology, waxing, manicures, and a makeover are much the same as treating a client in a salon, although the work is more intense and possibly more time consuming. This is because there are special issues involved when working with the frail and infirm.

The therapist needs to be aware that some clients may not be able to endure a long treatment. Be alert for any signs of distress or other changes that can occur during a treatment, and be able to handle an 'unexpected' situation when it arises. Experience and time will help the therapist cope with the many ever-challenging tasks that she may face.

In many frail persons there can be a wide range of skin complaints and some people may have a combination of them. What they have in common is that their skin can be very dry, mainly because of dehydration. Also heating or air conditioning systems will have an effect on the skin. Most clients in poor health can have continuing skin problems. This may also relate to poor nutrition and other aspects that I have mentioned. As the old saying goes, 'what goes in shows through the skin'. Clients in hostel accommodation can vary with skin conditions depending on their age, illness, their medication or nutritional intake. Not all is gloom and doom, as I have come across many older women who have lovely soft skin known as the 'English rose' complexion. These women have 'inherited' lovely skin and have looked after their skin properly all of their lives; their efforts have paid off.

For hostel care residents the therapist usually gives a facial or face reflexology with the client either sitting in a chair, or lying down on a bed. Some residents may be in a wheelchair. As I mentioned in Chapter 1, most nursing homes provide a room where a therapist can work. I have found the lighting often to be better in the home's salon than in a client's room. While treating the residents in the home's salon or community room, it is best to give treatment to a client sitting in a chair. The time spent giving a facial depends on how long the client can sit without getting restless. I have found the longest most clients can take is 20 to 30 minutes. In this time I am able to give a cleansing, exfoliation, a mask treatment and a face massage including face reflexology.

Possible options for shorter sessions might be:

- cleansing, exfoliation and a mask treatment

- cleansing, exfoliation and a face massage.

Most clients, however, will enjoy the full facial procedure.

This is where the therapist will use discretion in what is best for the client. The therapist may find that they may treat four women with a facial in one morning session, but find that each one will require a different routine. The main aim is to give the skin a good cleanse to help rejuvenate and moisten the skin, leaving the client feeling refreshed and comfortable. It is not so much a question of how long the therapy will take, it is more to do with the touch and the attention the person receives. Helping her to look and feel good will give her a sense of dignity and instils confidence. Focus on quality and care is most important.

WORKING AROUND BEDS, CHAIRS, WHEELCHAIRS AND LOUNGE CHAIRS

If a client is lying in a 'modern hospital' bed it is much easier to work. The bed can be raised to the right height for the therapist to work, and the bed ends will lift out. This makes it easier for the therapist to get behind the bed, to have the client's head close to the top end and for the therapist to be able to give treatment to the client without having to bend or stoop. Working from the chairs (ordinary or a wheelchair) can at times be a strain on the therapist's back, especially if the client constantly leans forward. In these cases it is best to limit the time. Lounge chairs are lower and I do not find it easy to give facials from this angle. I will ask the nursing staff or a carer to help move the client onto a bed. If the therapist can cope with the client sitting in the chair that is fine, but care must be taken of one's back.

BEFORE GIVING A FACIAL

Put on disposable gloves before commencing treatment. There are several possible reasons for needing gloves.

- The client is unable to eat properly and will dribble food crumbs which fall around the neck region or accumulate around the mouth and nose (the client may not have been washed before treatment).

- Dribbling (a common problem with some frail clients).

- Uncontrollable tongue movements may disrupt procedures.

- Spillage of fluids and liquid medication are some common mishaps.

- It is essential to observe hygiene regulations.

Frail clients can become restless or continue with involuntary movements if they have suffered either a stroke, heart condition, injury, or have Parkinson's disease, multiple sclerosis, dementia, or experience a reaction to the side effects of medication or are in pain. These involuntary movements can include:

- head tremors

- hand movements

- shaking

- rocking back and forwards in a chair

- facial movements

- eye squinting

- mouth movements.

If these movements intensify, it is best to stop and see what the client wants. Ask her if she needs assistance. If she cannot answer, stop the treatment. It may mean that the client is wanting to go to the rest room or that she needs to be changed or has the urge to wander. This is a common occurrence among clients with dementia. When situations like this arise, go to find a carer or a nurse to assist. With experience, the therapist will be able to 'body read' and see the signs which mean when to stop and when to continue with a restless client. Don't be put off by these challenges: they will only make you more aware of a client's needs and your ability to 'specialise' in such a challenging and rewarding environment.

Many of the conditions that I have mentioned can also occur with young disabled persons. Young persons may also reside in a nursing home or in hostel care and can have many of the same disorders of the skin, fingernails and toenails as I have found in frail older people. This may be due to their illness, medication, injuries and the inability to take care of their personal hygiene needs.

> On some occasions I have found, when working with clients who suffer with dementia, that they can become restless during a treatment if a familiar toy or object (ball, box, handkerchief, purse, etc.) is lost or taken from them. A special toy like a doll can be 'real' to them (like a small child or baby) and they can guard it as if they were looking after a child. I have found if one of my clients had a doll to nurse she would become more relaxed and communicate happily while having her treatment. On some occasions the client has asked me to give her 'baby' a face clean and I have been happy to do this. The therapist will get better results with a client's treatment if she incorporates the client's toy, object or animal into the session. If the toy or object has to be removed, make sure the client can see it and tell her it is okay for 'baby' to be there or that the ball, box, etc. is beside her and you will make sure no one else will take it away. Sense of security is very important to a client with dementia, no matter what it is to which she is attached.

A FACIAL FOR FRAIL PERSONS

Use a warm towel or a disposable face cloth to remove the dirt and continue with a cleanser. If a client continues to dribble or secrete any other fluid, it is best to keep wearing gloves, otherwise remove them after the first cleanse. Exfoliate the skin using your hands, any abrasive brush or rough sponges may be too harsh for the client's delicate skin, so manual stimulation is best. Once again assess the client's skin and comfort, and apply what is best for her. When applying a mask use one that is light and has more natural ingredients. Remove the mask and give a massage or face reflexology using essential oils or cosmetic creams. There is no need to bring in any salon machinery to use for vaporising or exfoliating. The therapist needs to remember that she is not going to achieve the same success in treating a frail client's skin as they would on a client in a salon. The main aim is to help the client's skin look clean, and for the client to feel good, leaving her feeling refreshed and comfortable after her treatment. Once the treatment is completed moisturiser cream should be applied to the skin. There is no need to put too much moisturiser on the skin after a facial, unless the client wishes to wear makeup.

> In most of the nursing homes I have visited, I have found that most carers and nursing staff have been very efficient in their work and are constantly attending to the residents' personal needs. However, there are times when nursing staff can be very busy attending to other residents. The therapist may turn up to give her client treatment before the staff have had the chance to prepare her. Some residents require ongoing attention for the reasons stated above and this may apply to the therapist's client. Sometimes there can be a staff shortage on the day of a visit, so it is important to be patient if nursing staff assistance is required. The other option is to postpone the client's appointment if the therapist finds her time is limited.

MAKEUP
The eyebrows and colour tints
Eyebrows on frail older people lose shape and the hairs can become wiry, coarse and grow long with grey or white strands. Some women have very few hairs left on their brows or sometimes none at all. If there are moles along the hairline, or near the eyebrow hairline, creating a smooth line can sometimes be difficult. For those who have only a few hairs I have found that an eyebrow tint will to do the trick. After a few treatments the colour picks up on the fine hairs along the brow line leaving a definite line in the shape of the brow, much to the satisfaction of the client. For long wiry hairs, I remove a few hairs but take care not to remove too many if no short hairs are present. Work with what is best for the client. This is where the therapist can act like a magician and create some 'form' so that a brow ends up looking a lot

better than before. Some women have very thick eyebrows and the hairs can be strong, with grey and white hairs mixed in with their own natural colour. Women who have thick brows generally like them thinned out, but not too thin. Removing hairs from thick eyebrows can be very painful and sometimes it can cause bleeding. Any bleeding with hair removal always necessitates the use of disposable gloves.

> Cutting eyebrow hairs is not always a good option as this can lead to the hairs becoming very coarse and producing abnormal regrowth.

Eyebrow tints

As mentioned above, some women benefit from an eyebrow colour tint, especially when the eyebrows have lost their natural colour and very few hairs are visible. The colour tint will pick up on fine hairs but will not adhere very well to coarse grey or white hairs.

> Never apply a colour tint to the eyebrow if the person has any problems relating to their eyes such as an eye disorder, infection, soreness, inflammation or sensitivity.

Eyelash tints

It is unlikely that the therapist will be asked to give an eyelash tint to a frail elderly woman. Due to the conditions I have mentioned, some elderly women no longer have many eyelashes left, however, on some occasions I have tinted eyelashes for young women who were in care.

Very few older women will wear mascara, due to mascara irritation and for the same reasons I have mentioned. Contaminated mascara wands can cause an infection to the eyes especially if the cornea of the eye is scratched by the mascara wand.

A therapist should never work near the eyes with any cosmetic treatment if the client shows any signs of:

- inflammation

- soreness

- swelling in the eyes or around the eyes

- watery eyes

- infections

- very loose skin over the eyelids or around the eyes

- blepharitis (an inflammation of the eyelids)

- other eye disorders.

Makeup application

Occasionally the therapist may be asked to do a makeover for a client who likes to wear makeup and for others who like to be made over for a special occasion. Most women who reside in a nursing home just require a basic touch of makeup so they can look and feel good. I found it is best to use lighter colours in foundation, and in colour application I use a matt texture. Dark colours emphasise wrinkles and can make the face look older, whereas lighter colours have the opposite effect, giving a more 'natural' look. There are a few women who remain in the 'era of their youth' and they will continue to wear makeup as they did when young. Unfortunately it is very difficult to get them to change their minds and to move them into the present time, showing them how the makeup of today would be more flattering. In situations like this, it is best to put new ideas aside and give them what they want. After all, they are not going to change and are very happy being as they are, which is what really matters. Younger women however, like to follow contemporary trends.

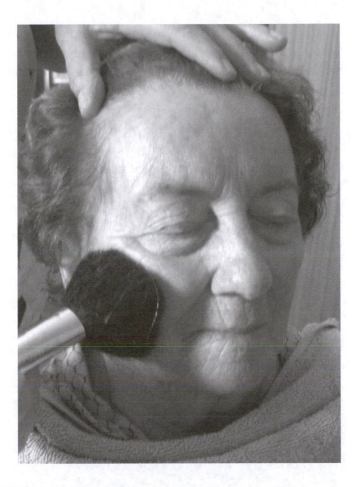

FIGURE 5.1 A powder brush is used to apply powder evenly over the client's face before light colour makeup is applied.

Makeup tips for older women

1. I use a *tinted moisturiser* and apply it all over the face. A light foundation can be applied, that is, if the client wants it. A neutral foundation with an SPF can also be another alternative. (Some women may insist on using their own foundation.)

2. *Apply loose powder* in a blotting motion using a disposable cotton pad, followed by a powder brush to achieve a natural matte finish to the skin (Figure 5.1). The face is now ready for the colour makeup. In some cases the client will only want these two steps finished off with lipstick. (The basic step.)

The new *mineral powders* on the market today can be a substitute for the above. Apply as for step 2, this will give a better coverage than just using the powder brush.

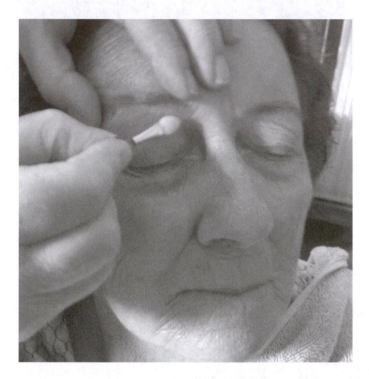

FIGURE 5.2 The therapist applies a light coloured eye shadow to the client's eyelids and under the eyebrow line.

3. For *extra colour* (women who like to have a little colour on the eyelids), I will add powder, blusher and some light eye shadow colour to the eyes (Figure 5.2). In many frail elderly women I have found it is not always advisable to apply eye shadow to the eyelids. This is mainly due to some of the problems previously mentioned. Women who can wear colour shadow will only need a little highlight under

the brow and over the eyelid area. A neutral or soft pastel colour can be added over the eyelid to help accentuate the eyes. I rarely use an eye pencil or any form of shadow underneath the eye as this may easily lead to irritations, infections and discomfort. Blusher can be added either before lipstick or after. It is not necessary to use a blusher or rouge on an elderly woman if her skin is highly coloured.

4. *For the eyebrows*, I use a brow brush with a touch of eye shadow colour adding to the hairs of the eyebrow, giving the brows a natural look. If I use a pencil, I may use two colours such as a grey and a light brown. I work along the brow line drawing in a feather motion to give an appearance of a natural eyebrow line. This is a good method for clients who have no visible eyebrow hairs.

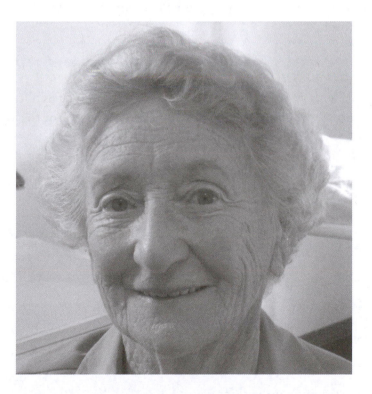

FIGURE 5.3 The client is pleased to have her eyebrows pencilled in along her eyebrow line, showing a natural colour.

5. *Lipstick is added last.* Powder lips using a cotton pad, then remove excess powder using a powder brush before adding the lipstick. After application of lipstick, blot the lips with a tissue to remove excess. Repeat this cycle two to three times as this helps to set the lipstick and it will last longer. Sometimes it is difficult to apply lipstick on some client's lips due to dribbling, uncontrollable lip movements, sucking in lips, or having very thin lips and numerous folds. For these women it would not be practical to apply lipstick. Powdering the lips using a disposable cotton pad will also help prevent lipstick 'bleeding'. For some elderly women it is not practical to use lip liner pencils. Blotting the lipstick will also help prevent lipstick adhering to the teeth.

Younger women in care will probably enjoy the benefits of a full makeover.

Sensitive skin

People with very sensitive skin can react to a cosmetic application as soon as the cosmetic is applied to the skin. Some of the signs may be:

- coughing
- sneezing
- watery eyes
- stinging eyes
- breathing difficulties
- runny nose
- skin turning a slight pink to very red
- skin going blotchy with pink or red spots
- stinging on the skin
- itching.

Should a person show any of these signs remove the offending cosmetic immediately. You may apply a cool compress to reduce any inflammation.

> Calendula infusion makes a wonderful compress as it works quickly to resolve any inflammation of the skin. The calendula oil is as effective as a herbal infusion. Clients may also react to strong fragrances and this is one of the reasons why I do not wear perfume while I am attending to clients, either in my salon or outside on location.

The counting method

(These are tips I gave to a woman who was blind from birth.) Millie (not her real name) always wanted to know how to wear makeup. She said she felt she had missed out on doing things like other girls, especially in her youth. Millie said that she only wanted to feel what it was like to wear makeup and know how to apply it. After being with her, I went home to my salon and sat down to reflect on a plan that would be easy for Millie to follow. I blindfolded myself and came up with an idea of 'counting' and feeling the cosmetics. I imagined that I was touching the cosmetics for the first time and how I would apply my moisturiser, powder, blusher and lipstick. When I practised this method a few times I soon found the solution that would suit my client. This is what I did:

MOISTURISER

Once I managed to remove the lid off my moisturiser jar, I took a spatula and some cream. Next I took the cream from the spatula and placed it on my thumbnail so I could feel how much cream I needed to apply to my face. This gave me an idea of whether I had enough to place all over my face and neck. Taking the cream from my thumbnail, I placed dots over my cheeks, nose, chin and forehead using my index finger. Then I gently rubbed the cream evenly into the skin with my fingers. I continued rubbing until I felt that all the cream had absorbed into my skin.

FACE POWDER

Using a compact powder, I placed a powder brush over the powder and after three long strokes, I then placed the brush over my wrist and gave the brush two gentle hits to remove any excess powder from the brush. Next I placed the powder brush over my cheeks, lips and forehead (the eyes were omitted) and I spread it evenly over my face and lips, counting three times with each stroke as I worked in a circular motion.

BLUSHER APPLICATION

Taking a blusher brush, I felt my cheek bones with my fingers and then I placed the brush into the blusher. I gave three gentle taps with the brush over my wrist to remove any excess powder and in an upward stroke I placed the brush over my right cheek counting three times, and then I repeated the same sequence on my left cheek.

LIPSTICK APPLICATION

The way that I thought would be best for Millie was to place the lipstick from the tube directly to the lips. First I ran my fingers over my lip-line to get the feel of how wide my lips are. Then I felt the length of the lipstick, after partially screwing it out of its container. I placed the lipstick along my lips slowly and carefully. Using a tissue I blotted away any excess lipstick. I also used a tissue to clean my lipstick tube after I had applied it.

These actions took me a few lessons before I could master them blindfolded and was confident to try them on my client. At first it was trial and error and it took a few sessions before she could feel confident to apply some of the cosmetics. The moisturiser and powder were easy to use and we concentrated on this until she was ready to try blusher and lipstick. Once Millie had mastered cosmetic application, she felt confident to wear it sometimes when she went out with friends. She was delighted to have experienced the feel of using makeup and I had the satisfaction of knowing that I had succeeded in giving something 'special' to a client who had missed out on so much when it came to cosmetics and beauty therapy.

WAXING FOR OLDER WOMEN
Facial hair problems

Unwanted hair growth has always been a problem for every age group but methods of hair removal have been equally problematic. Dealing with facial hair, in particular, among older women has caused embarrassment and discomfort. There are many factors that may cause unwanted hair growth. These could be:

- taking certain medications

- hormonal changes (increased dihydrotestosterone (DHT) during menopause is another reason hair on the face goes from fine to coarse)

- genetic disorders

- using chemical-based creams

- shaving.

Some clients may not have had facial hair problems until later in life. This could mean that the client has:

- changed to another medication

- a hormonal imbalance

- an illness that has progressed, causing the hair growth

- a carer who had started shaving her.

Some women may need waxing more often than others because their hair growth is faster, which may be due to a change in hormones, illness or medication. The hair continues to grow strongly at the same length as it was before the last waxing. There is not a lot a therapist can do, only give the quality of care, and allow the client some comfort between appointments. If the client is able to continue with the waxing, it is best for her, because the skin feels smoother after waxing, with no consequences of ingrown hairs or roughness, as is found with shaving. Other forms of removing hair would not be practical to use on frail clients. Women who continue to use depilatory creams can end up with skin problems such as:

- skin burning

- skin rashes

- blisters

- scarring.

If a chemical in a cream can damage hard keratin in hair, then it is able to burn and damage sensitive skin. Never use any hair removal cream on a frail person. Bleaching hairs on the face similarly can cause problems to the skin. This is another method used by some women to disguise unwanted hair. In my view waxing is probably the best method if the client can cope with the treatment. Older women who have lesions or sores accumulating from skin cancers can cope with a cold strip wax. The wax must not be applied more than once over any area of the skin or applied near any visible lesion or sores. Never wax if the sores are inflamed, bleeding or weepy.

> I am always amazed how many women can put up with hair removal by waxing. As one older client told me, she was in so much pain with her other body parts that waxing was nothing compared to what she was suffering daily. Another reason can be that some older frail clients can loose nerve sensation in the face and do not feel the hairs being removed, especially if the hairs are fine.

Over a period of time when the client has had regular waxing, the hairs will grow back very thin and are easily removed with little discomfort to the client. On other occasions I had to cease waxing a client because the hair was too coarse and strong to remove from a delicate skin. Removing coarse hair from delicate skin can cause bleeding and inflammation; this causes the client too much pain, therefore, in these circumstances it is best to leave things as they are.

Methods for safe waxing

For safety and hygiene reasons I found it was not practical to take a hot wax pot into a nursing home. Not only did I find it time consuming but hot wax and warm wax on frail clients can be a painful experience for them and the wax can easily cause burns, due to their skin thinness and sensitivity. Trying to warm up the wax takes time, and a safe place for the pot to stand is not always available. The main safety factor is trying to find a place to warm up wax, which is out of the way of wandering residents, especially those who have dementia. Special rooms or a salon are not always available in a nursing home. Usually I have to give a client a wax treatment in her room and this can be more difficult with hot wax as there is little room for safe placement of the pot.

If hot or warm wax is not an option, what should the therapist use? Today there are many wax products on the market that don't need to be kept warm in a wax pot. There are cold waxes where you just take the wax from the jar and apply it direct to the 'hairy' area and remove with a strip. These waxes sound ideal and would be great for using in hotter climates, but I have found them to be useless as they become hard in cooler climates and impractical to use. There are some waxes that require warming up in a microwave oven, which is probably alright if you are working from one room, as in a nursing home's beauty salon. However, this is very time consuming for one-to-one room service, especially if you have to run around to find an available microwave oven and then monitor the heat and safe passage back to the client's room. The best form of wax I have used over the years when I visit frail clients is cold wax strips (Figure 5.4). I use a brand that supplies the wax in a box of 12 strips, each wax sheet has two cellophane strips that can be pulled apart and both sides can be used. They work well and have the same function as any hot or warm wax. The wax strips are all disposable and are easy to cut to the exact strip size needed. There are many brands available, so it is best to choose one that will be suitable for use on frail persons. Not all cold wax strips are as good as claimed, because some of them do not adhere adequately to the unwanted hair. The other disadvantages are that cold waxes do not always take all the hairs in one sweep like the warm and hot wax, and the strip wax can become very sticky, especially in hot weather. New varieties of wax are constantly coming on the market, so I suggest the therapist keeps in touch with any improved products that could be beneficial for her older clients.

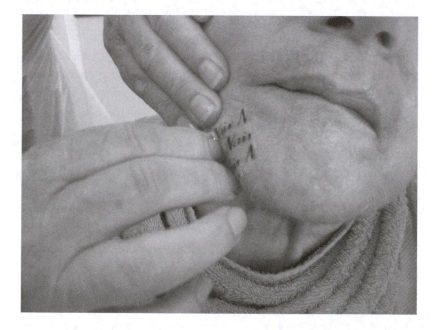

FIGURE 5.4 Using disposable wax strips is a better alternative to using a hot wax or warm wax when visiting a client at home, in a nursing home, in hospital or in palliative care.

Caution with waxing

Some cold wax strips and other waxes do have ingredients that can be harmful on skins of the frail elderly, such as those who suffer with diabetes, circulatory problems and skin problems. Examples of the latter include:

- varicose veins

- moles

- warts

- eczema and psoriasis

- sensitive skin

- damaged skin.

Due to these conditions, some women are not good candidates for waxing. For those who are able to have a waxing treatment, choose the strips that are effective without too many harmful ingredients.

> In my experience I have found the clear wax strips I have used have proved successful on the majority of frail women, leaving them with no trauma, apart from the 'usual' redness on some.

Waxing facial hair

The main two areas that a therapist will be asked to wax on the face are the chin and across the top lip. If waxing a client for the first time, use disposable gloves because the client's skin may bleed, especially if the hairs are strong and coarse. Start on a patch of hair from the side of the face. This is the testing stage to see how the client will cope with the waxing. If she protests too much, the test patch won't look too out of place on the face if she is unable to continue. Full facial waxes are sometimes asked for. This generally includes the chin, top lip, sides of the face and sometimes the neck. Younger women in care, may ask for a leg wax or a bikini wax. Depending on the disability of the person, and providing they can cope, the therapist may need to ask a carer or member of the nursing staff to assist in helping to manoeuvre the client into different positions for the waxing treatment if the client's mobility is poor.

> The therapist must be careful when waxing the top lip of frail older women. This is because most frail women have very thin lips and the skin can tear easily with waxing. I have found it best to wax across the top lip just above the lip line and a little below the nose. For the remaining hairs left around the corner of the mouth, it is best to remove them with tweezers.

MANICURE TIPS

Basic steps in a manicure

This service will possibly take the therapist longer than any other beauty service for a person in care. This is because the cleaning of fingernails, and preparing for the client's needs, requires detailed care and attention. The basic manicure procedure is probably enough for frail people. This comprises:

- cleansing
- removing of any old varnish
- fingernail cutting (if necessary)
- filing the nails
- cuticle care
- cleaning the fingernails, around the cuticles and under the nails
- fingernail shaping
- buffing
- using nail coating
- colour varnish.

(The last two are optional.)

> Care is needed when cutting across the free-edge of the fingernail when giving a manicure to a frail older person. I have

found if I held my supporting finger across the fingerpad of the person receiving the treatment, I would gently pull away the fingerpad from the free-edge of the nail as this prevents nicking any loose skin. In my experience it is best to use nail scissors instead of nail clippers. Nail clippers will tear the nail if the fingernails are thin, brittle or very thick.

Once the therapist has established how they are going to work over, or around, their client and attend to their needs, treatment can begin. Working on a client sitting in a wheelchair, lying on a lounge chair, sitting at a table, or lying in a bed, are all suitable positions for giving a manicure. For props I use a pillow with a clean towel over the pillow so she can rest her hands if she is in bed, sitting in a lounge chair or wheelchair with a tray attached. This makes it easier to work on the fingernails and it provides comfort. If the client sits at a table, I would use a small pillow and a clean towel, as when working from a manicure table in my salon. With clients who have suffered a stroke, I would put a hand roll in the palm of the client's affected hand. (A hand roll can be made by rolling a hand towel or face washer in a roll resembling a long sausage and big enough for the fingers to separate and fit comfortably over the roll, giving room to work on the nails.) This method works well when giving a client hand reflexology.

Step guide to a basic manicure

1. *Remove any old nail varnish* from the nail using a non-acetone varnish remover (acetone in nail varnish remover strips the nail of its natural oils, which may cause the nail to dry and flake) (Figure 5.5).

2. *Cleansing the hands and fingernails.* Put on disposable gloves and have the client soak their hands in a bowl of warm water with an antiseptic cleanser. If the client is unable to put her hands in a bowl, soak a towel and place the antiseptic cleanser on the towel and give the hands a 'sponge' bath. I use a tea-tree cleanser as it has good antiseptic properties. Make sure all dirt is removed from the hands. Stroke

victims can often have a strong odour coming from the affected hand, which is moist and an ideal area for fungi to grow. The fingernails are often weak on this hand as well, so go gently when working this area. However, because of the constant use of their stronger hand, the fingernails collect dirt and sometimes there are traces of faecal matter underneath the fingernails. Continue using disposable gloves until all cleansing is finished. In some cases you will need to keep gloves on all through the manicure. For very stubborn dirt I have found using the essential nail oils helpful. (See Chapter 6, 'Natural Therapies for Older People'.)

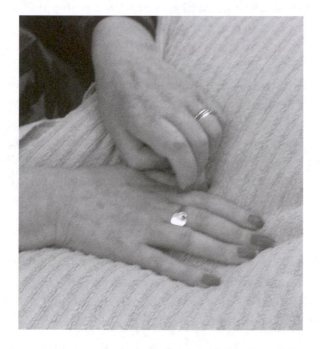

FIGURE 5.5 The client's nails have been painted a dark colour; this leaves the nails discoloured. The therapist removes the coloured varnish to allow 'breathing space' for the nails to rejuvenate.

Make sure the fingernails and fingers are dried thoroughly. Water will weaken frail fingernails, which may easily split when cut or filed.

3. *Cutting the free-edge of fingernails.* Cutting the nails to file and shape is quick and easy. Cut across the free-edge of the nail (or use a coarse file for thick nails) but do not cut corners on the nail as this may lead to infection (Figure 5.6). Some fingernails can be very strong and difficult to cut. Never try to cut strong coarse nails: use a rough nail file to shape the nail, then use a fine file to smooth rough edges.

Only cut the nail if necessary. With some agitated women, cutting the nail and filing is a quicker option to complete the treatment. Never use nail clippers as I have found them to be unsafe: when used on frail women, the skin on top of their fingers has very little subcutaneous tissue. The tips of the fingers can become very sensitive and if the nail is too thick or thin the nail clipper may rip the free-edge away, taking more nail than necessary. If this occurs, the client may be vulnerable to infections.

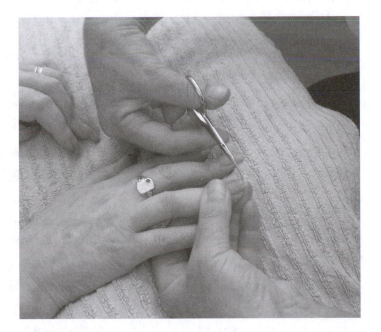

FIGURE 5.6 The therapist cuts across the free-edge of the fingernail on the client's hand slightly pulling back her finger pad (top of finger) to prevent cutting the skin.

4. *To clean around the fingernail, and underneath the nail.* Sometimes these areas will house stubborn dirt (and sometimes faecal matter). Dirt can be very difficult to remove and time consuming. I have found the best way to remove 'dirt matter' from underneath the nail is to use a cotton bud dipped in vegetable-based oil and applied underneath the nails for a few minutes. Another method is to apply the oil from an eye dropper allowing the oil to drop underneath the free-edge of each finger and thumbnail. The oil will loosen the stubborn dirt and you can easily lift out the dirt with a cuticle stick which can be disposed of after use. Use the oil around the nail fold to remove any other remaining dirt. The oil can be used to remove dead skin underneath the nail causing less discomfort for the client. Generally carers are responsible for removing any stubborn dirt from nails but in most cases I have found nails in need of proper cleaning. Some clients are ultra-sensitive to touch underneath the nail, and this is where the oil application makes it easier for the client to cope with cleaning procedures.

5. *Once the dirt has been removed,* cleanse the hands and fingers once again.

6. *Apply cuticle remover* in the form of cuticle remover liquids, creams or nail oils. This helps loosen the dead skin around the cuticles and nail fold.

7. *Leave the cuticle remover* on each finger and thumb for a few minutes before removing the dead skin from around the cuticles and nail fold.

8. *Remove your gloves* and give your hands a full cleanse. Use a new pair of disposable gloves (if necessary).

9. *Shape the fingernails.* It is easy to follow the line of the nail, and most clients prefer rounded or oval. Younger clients may like the pointed shape or whatever shape is fashionable but, really, apart from the round or oval, other shapes may not be practical.

10. *Use a white pencil under the free-edge* of the fingernails to camouflage stains; it does make a difference. (Make sure the pencil is sharpened before each use.)

    Liquid whitener may be too strong to use on frail persons.

11. *Remove any dead skin from the cuticle area* by gently scraping the dead skin away from the cuticle and nail fold, using a disposable cuticle stick or a reusable stainless steel instrument (Figure 5.7). Carefully push the cuticles down if the skin around the cuticles has grown up on to the nail plate. (This can be very painful to the client, therefore judge if it is worth taking any further steps in cuticle treatment.) Using nail oils or cream may help soften the cuticles.

    Never try to force abnormal cuticle skin growth down the fingernail, especially on a frail elderly person as the pressure may cause the skin to break, and bleeding may occur around the cuticle, which may lead to an infection.

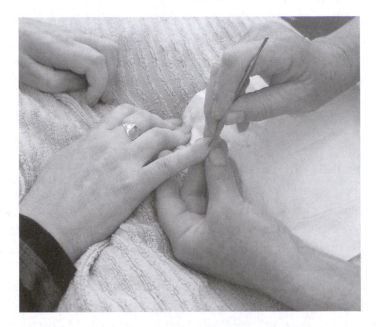

FIGURE 5.7 The therapist gently scrapes away the dead skin around the client's cuticles making sure not to cause damage to the skin.

12. *Apply cuticle oils* or cream for strengthening and nourishment to the nails and for cuticle treatment. The oils or cream will soften any loose skin around the cuticle, which makes it easier to remove at a later stage. If the oils are unsuitable to use on your client, use a cuticle cream. Work the oil or cream around the nail, over the cuticles and under the free-edge with circular movements.

I use my own nail oil treatment, made from a mixture of base and essential oils, which I have found to be beneficial for the cuticles and nails.

13. *Remove any excess oil or cream* with a clean tissue and lightly buff the nails with a soft smooth buffing file.

14. *Apply hand cream to hands* and the forearm and give a massage, as most people respond enthusiastically. (Hand reflexology may be given at this stage.)

15. *Apply clear varnish* to the fingernails followed by a clear varnish. If the client wants colour, apply this after a base coat and before the top coat or clear varnish.

If using essential oil for nail treatment, there is no need to apply nail varnish after the manicure. Some clients may have an allergy to nail varnish, therefore the use of cosmetic and essential oils, cosmetic cream and buffing may be enough.

Coloured nail varnish (or polish)

It is best to use nail colours that are quick drying. Painting the fingernails with colour can be very time consuming because some clients, due to restlessness, or uncontrollable twitches, are unable to keep their hands still. It takes a lot of skill and patience to overcome these obstacles. Do not apply colour varnish if the client's nails are discoloured; allow the nails to have 'breathing space' and see what the cause of the discoloration may be. Sometimes constant use of nail colour is the main reason for nail discoloration, and leaving the nails free from colour for a few weeks can make a big difference.

As a student in beauty therapy, I was taught that it is not a good idea to cut nails, only file them. Giving a manicure to an older person in care is not always practical due to time and discomfort for the person receiving treatment. Some residents can be restless all through their treatment and the therapist will need to work carefully and quickly. However, there are damaged nails, as in 'ram's horn', which are very difficult to cut and I would advise not to try. With so many new files on the market today, there are a few coarse files that are suitable for filing thick nails. I have found that older clients do not like to have long fingernails. Sometimes this can become a problem as some are adamant that they want their nails very short. Trying to explain that having very short nails is not good for the nail, and can lead to infections and other nail problems, does not seem to register with some people. Also, constantly cutting fingernails short frequently can weaken the nails causing splitting and frayed edging. With a lot of perseverance and patience, I have managed to persuade some women at least to let the nail grow up towards the free-edge.

If the client is holding something, work on one hand at a time and transfer the toy or object to the other hand. Do this if the client does not want to let it go. Never let a client become agitated or upset if they find comfort with whatever they may be holding. This scenario is common among clients who have dementia.

CHAPTER 6

Natural Therapies for Older People

WHAT IS NATURAL THERAPY?

Natural therapy is a term used to describe a variety of ancient traditional medicine that has been passed down through the ages. In the twentieth century it has regained its popularity and is recognised as complementary medicine that has proved to be beneficial alongside some conventional medical treatments. Natural therapies are often referred to as holistic medicine, alternative medicine and complementary medicine. There is a range of therapies that are used in conjunction with conventional treatments, such as naturopathy, herbal medicine, acupuncture, acupressure, homeopathy, iridology, massage, aromatherapy, osteopathy, reflexology and reiki. The healing power of nature is the principle with which every natural therapist is familiar, and they employ various methods of treatment compatible with this 'vital' curative activity of the body to stimulate and potentiate homeostatic mechanisms.

'Health is wholeness', and holistic medicine is the treatment of the whole person. Each person is unique, and cannot be labelled with a particular diagnosis and then the assumption made that this label contains all relevant information about them. Each person needs to be viewed as a person with a problem, of which the sickness is but a manifestation. Treatments should be tailored to the particular person. What is right for one is not necessarily right for another, even though the disease may be the same (Southern Cross Herbal School 1997, pp.3, 4, 7).

Natural therapies offer an abundance of relevant, valid techniques, reflecting the diversity of human consciousness.

Whether looking to ease aching muscles, relieving a cold, soothing the stress of an ulcer or bathing sore eyes, there are therapies and modalities to suit every condition and person. Emphasis is on assisting people to understand and help themselves, with education on self-care rather than dependence, and clients taking responsibility for their own health is encouraged by many natural therapists.

The use of natural therapies is becoming very popular, especially in nursing homes and other aged care centres, as well as for palliative care. When I visit a nursing home, I see certain therapies such as massage, aromatherapy, reflexology, and Tai Chi being introduced to the residents. These therapies have been embraced by many older people. The main incentive for incorporating natural therapies for an older person is to help them to feel good, to encourage relaxation and to instil a sense of well-being into their daily health care, so that there is 'acceptance' of the benefits the therapy may give. Up until 18 years ago, reflexology was not familiar to many older persons and it was considered 'quack medicine', along with other natural therapies that have evolved in recent years. The generation of my parents and grandparents were dubious about the different therapies that were offered to them. When I began as a 'novice' therapist I visited various homes giving talks and demonstrations to the residents, introducing my modalities of beauty therapy, massage, aromatherapy and reflexology. From these talks and demonstrations, I attracted a few clients for initial trials. Over a period of time, many clients became familiar with these therapies and looked forward to their fortnightly treatment. Visits from other natural therapists have also been valuable to the residents. Older people like to receive touch, so therapies that involve body work are more likely to be requested. Touch and the quality of care are important with older persons and younger persons in care, as these therapies help them to feel good, and they enjoy having 'one-to-one' special attention from the therapist.

This is the main focus when giving treatment to a frail or a disabled person. Progress may be very slow in achieving positive results in frail older persons and those in palliative care. However, there are positive forms of healing taking place, as the body will respond in some way, if not physically, then certainly on a spiritual and emotional level. While a client is continuing with regular treatment, it is a good sign that she may feel a change within her whole being; this is considered 'positive' progress.

> In my experience I have found that the most positive outcome in giving a treatment in natural therapy on a frail person is that her attitude can change for the better. She is able to come to terms with her illness or disability, and be more at peace with herself.

INTRODUCING NATURAL THERAPIES TO A CLIENT

While some clients may enjoy the touch of a massage or reflexology, they may not understand what the benefits are, and often get confused thinking that the therapy may help cure them. As a therapist, it is important to explain to a client how the therapy works and how it may benefit her. Although the therapy may prove to be successful in treating some conditions, it is best to focus on the 'relaxation' and helping the client feel good after treatment. If the therapy has helped with her ailments, this is a bonus. Some frail people may be very vulnerable and open to any kind of treatment in the hope that it may cure or improve their condition. The therapist must take care in the management of how to handle a vulnerable person. On the other hand, there are clients who are realistic in the knowledge that their ailments are not going to be cured, and that any therapy which can alleviate pain or discomfort, even for a short period of time, is better than receiving no treatment at all.

When introducing a therapy to the client, the therapist should explain exactly what she is going to do, and what the client may feel during and after the treatment. For her first session it is best not give a long treatment, just enough that the person can feel comfortable, adjusting to the therapy and getting used to the therapist's touch. After a few treatments, depending on her frailty, the client may be able to have a longer session. Don't 'overstimulate' a frail client with body therapies as she can become very tired and exhausted, especially if she is not used to touch. I have found older persons who have had body therapies previously will adapt easily to body therapy treatment.

> Over the years, I have seen a few therapists visit aged-care homes to give a client a massage. Although these therapists worked with the best of intentions, a few of them made mistakes in their dealings with their clients and were not asked back to the home. Some mistakes listed below were recounted to me by my clients and carers.
>
> Examples are:
>
> - the frail client had difficulty in trying to get onto the massage table
>
> - the therapist did not assess the client properly and worked on her with too heavy a touch (in some instances caused bruising)
>
> - the therapist was a new graduate with little experience in working with frail people
>
> - time-consuming factors for the therapist, that is, the therapist underestimated client mobility, time in preparation and so completion time took longer
>
> - the therapist was unable to cope with the client's condition
>
> - the session was too tiring for the client.

In this chapter I am not going to discuss all body therapies, only those that I practise, and some other holistic therapies which are currently very popular for use in nursing homes. Natural therapies, like the beauty industry, are growing into 'big business' and more people are using natural therapies, along with conventional medicine, to help maintain a healthy body and mind. Natural therapies will be used widely in the near future, especially as the 'baby boomers' are reaching their retirement, and this will be the generation that will demand such services. In the near future I would hope more trained therapists, working with older and frail persons, continue with complementary therapies as this would add to the client's quality of care, bringing a much more relaxed and peaceful tranquillity into her daily life.

The following sections simply provide guidelines in how best to use natural therapies when dealing with frail clients.

MASSAGE FOR OLDER PERSONS

Massage is primarily a technique of relaxation. It is an umbrella term used to describe the different modalities of massage and their different techniques. For example, Swedish, remedial, Bowen, shiatsu and acupressure are applied with differing pressure and hand movements, but each modality is aimed to help in the relief of stress and tension, the improvement of circulation and lymphatic flow. Massage can open the channels of communication between a client and a massage therapist, promoting contact on a physical and mental level.

A frail client is often very sensitive to touch and may take longer to adapt to the technique of a massage, especially if it is her first time. This may be due to:

- a bony prominence

- thinness of the skin

- the hypersensitivity of the skin

- swelling

- tightness in muscle tissue

- very little support of adipose (fat) tissue

- ill health factors

- tendency to bruising.

Swedish massage (a relaxing massage) with its soft flowing movements, and perhaps a Bowen treatment, is probably what most frail older people may cope with. Other modalities such as acupressure, aromatherapy, feet, hands and face reflexology, colour imaging and creative visualisation are some other therapies that can be incorporated with a relaxing massage. When working with frail clients, the therapist should always be guided by her intuition. 'Read' the body, looking for obvious indicators such as the sensitivities listed above or other non-verbal signs, so the therapist can estimate what the person can cope with in any particular session. Take into consideration that during an assessment the therapist may find that the client is not suitable for a massage, even though she may wish to continue.

PREPARING FOR A MASSAGE

I have found it best to give the client a massage lying in her own bed, providing that the bed is high enough for the therapist to easily manoeuvre around it. The new hospital beds are ideal for this. I have never taken a massage table into a nursing home or to a client's home, as most of them have been too frail to get on to the table themselves, and it is not feasible or safe to move the client into different positions or try to lift them. Although the hospital beds are wider than a massage table, the results are as effective giving a massage to a client as if she were lying on a massage table. I found these beds safer for the client because they are easier to manoeuvre into high or low positions.

> Previously some of these beds had side rails as a safety precaution to help prevent some frail residents from falling out of bed. Over time, these proved to be harmful as some residents were found to have arm or leg injuries and the rails had to be removed. The latest idea is to make sure the bed is kept very low and that gym mats are placed on the floor on both sides of the bed to protect the resident in case of a fall. Ideas are changing frequently, so the therapist needs to know what procedures to take when treating a frail client in their bed. Never leave a client unattended, especially if there is no protection of bed rails or gym mats and the bed has been raised. If you need to

leave the room during a client's treatment, ring for assistance. When the client's treatment is finished, make sure the bed is lowered and that the client can safely get in and out of the bed. This is an important issue when it comes to wandering clients with dementia. Always let the RN or carer know when you have finished with a client.

Before massage, ask the carer or nursing staff to place the client onto the bed. In some homes that I have visited, the client had been showered by the carers and put in the bed ready for my visit. This saved a lot of time. I found it was a good idea for me to arrange the client's appointment times with the nursing staff so they could have the client ready before I arrived. Some clients are able to dress and undress themselves and get on and off the bed without any problems. However, this can be very time consuming if the client has poor mobility, and there is not a lot you can do to speed things up, so it is best to be patient. It is important to encourage older people to do as much as they can for themselves; this allows them some sense of independence.

Older people feel the cold even in hot weather as many have poor circulation. Cover them with blankets and place towels over the covers so that oil or cream does not spill on to the blankets. Keep the client warm at all times, but do not cause the client to become 'overheated'. Take note of any skin lesions, bumps, bruises and other related skin problems and document details in a client's report file. If the client becomes a regular customer, the therapist will be able to notice if there are any positive or negative changes. If there are any changes that warrant concern, report them to the RN in charge.

MASSAGE TO THE HEAD, NECK AND SHOULDERS

Depending on the mobility of the client, it may be best to massage her while she is sitting in a chair rather than lying on the bed. Over the years I have given a massage to many clients seated in chairs, as this has been more comfortable for them while gently massaging around the neck, head and shoulder regions. It is not necessary to undress a client as the client can be massaged with part of her clothing removed and replaced after the massage. If the massage does not require any creams or oils, it is not necessary to remove clothing. Bowen therapy does not necessitate the removal of clothing as does Swedish or remedial massage. Always respect the client and allow her some dignity. In some cases, I have found that I can give a shoulder massage to a client without removing clothing. With the client's permission, I have gently massaged the shoulders underneath her clothing, placing a disposable cloth or towel around the top part of her blouse or dress to prevent cream or oil absorption into the clothing.

> Remember to place a towel over any 'exposed' areas so the client is not exposed to the elements. Another tip: I have found older people can have loose skin due to a loss of adipose tissue and muscle shrinkage. When massaging, I found it best to gently stretch the loose skin away from the area I was treating, and using gentle movements I could massage easily without causing friction to the skin or aggravation to any loose skin.

> People who have lost a considerable amount of weight can have layers of 'sagging' skin and the therapist needs to be very gentle when massaging around loose skin. Skin folds of loose skin can become inflamed by the aggravation; friction between the folds of skin rubbing together not only causes the skin to break, it can cause bruising, leading to an infection. This can be very uncomfortable and painful for the client.

If the therapist is going to massage a client sitting in a chair, it is best to make sure the client is comfortable and that the chair is not too low that it can cause the therapist to stoop or bend while working (Figure 6.1). If the chair is too low, ask the carer to transfer the client to a higher chair or on to the bed. Before commencing the massage, make sure the client's needs are met, especially if she needs to be cleaned or toileted.

The therapist should always be careful with their back while working with clients. A minor backache can develop into more serious problems later, if the therapist continues to stoop and bend while treating clients. Under no circumstances should a therapist try to lift a client onto a bed or into a chair. Always ask for assistance. Most nursing homes have a 'safety' policy for lifting and manoeuvring frail residents. Leave lifting up to the nursing staff or carers.

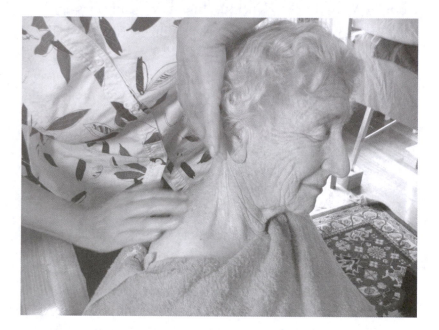

FIGURE 6.1 The client has a neck massage while sitting in a chair. Towels are used to prevent stains from essential oils or creams and to keep the client warm. The therapist slightly stretches the skin to prevent aggravation to loose skin.

MASSAGING THE LEGS AND FEET, ARMS AND HANDS

I have found that the best place to massage a client is to have her lying in, or on top of her bed where she can be more relaxed. The therapist can use any props that are required for a particular limb or body part. In my experience, most frail clients find a 30-minute session or even 20 minutes long enough. Older persons who are independent and more mobile are able to enjoy a longer session without any inhibitions. Once again assessment for each client will indicate how long, and what methods, she can cope with.

> While visiting some clients, especially on home visits, I have given a leg or arm massage while the client was sitting in a chair (Figures 6.2 and 6.3). For the legs and feet I would sit opposite her and have her legs on my lap, supported by a pillow with a towel covering the pillow, and additional support underneath her legs, such as a chair or a small table with more pillows or cushions covered with towels. This has worked well for both the client and for me. I have found this is a better alternative if the client is unable to get on to a bed or massage table, and her bed has been too low for me to work on.

> Massaging a client's arms and hands, I have found it best to have her sitting in a chair or wheelchair opposite me with a pillow placed between my lap and hers with a towel over the pillow. This helps the client to feel comfortable and relaxed. Extra support of pillows or towel rolls may help if necessary. Should the client be lying in or on the bed, I will use props such as towels and extra pillows for support to the arms and hands.

> The skin over the hands can also be loose, it is easier to gently pull the fingers downwards as if the client's hand was making a fist, or the therapist could move the skin to the side of the hand or down towards the fingers holding the skin with the fingers and massaging the client's hand with thumb movements, especially if the client is unable to follow instructions (Figure 6.3).

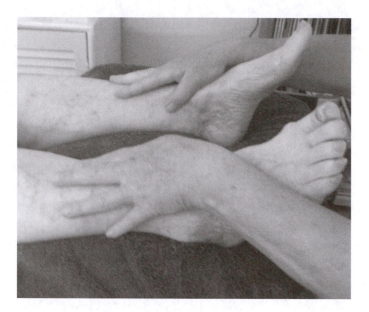

FIGURE 6.2 Leg massage can be relaxing for a frail client using gentle strokes with soft flowing movements.

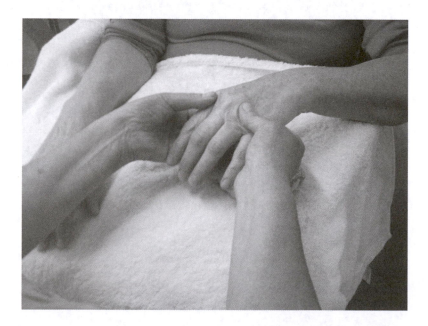

FIGURE 6.3 Hand massage is applied to a client who is sitting in a wheelchair. A pillow is used as a prop with a towel placed over the pillow.

GIVING A FULL BODY MASSAGE TO AN OLDER PERSON

It is very unlikely that a massage therapist will give full body treatments to frail older persons, especially for those who are in high care. However, there are exceptions, if the client previously had massage as part of their medical treatment. I have found that a full body massage is mostly requested by hostel and unit residents.

Older clients can find it difficult to manoeuvre themselves on the bed and to get into a comfortable position. If the client has poor or slow movements she can become stressed and exhausted. For such clients who have difficulty, it is easier for the therapist to manage the best they can, and work to the areas of the body that are easily accessible. Some clients can roll onto their sides, making it easier to massage their back. Massage one side and then get her to roll on to the other side. For hygiene and protection, when giving a client a full body massage always ensure that she has clean underwear, and keep her covered with blankets and clean towels for extra warmth. If the client is lying in 'soiled' linen do not proceed; get the carer to attend to her before the commencement of treatment. It is important that a client can feel clean and refreshed; she is more likely to relax and not feel uncomfortable if she has been attended to. Accidents do happen, and not only with older persons; they can happen with younger people in care, as well as those in palliative care. It is important to instil some dignity when a client has an 'unexpected' mishap.

USING ESSENTIAL OILS

Unless the therapist is a trained herbalist or aromatherapist, I suggest applying the basics for external application, base oils and essential oils for all body work on the frail. For some older clients the use of essential oils is contraindicated, therefore a massage cream or the client's own cream is a better alternative.

There are many essential oils on the market today with a wide range of fragrances and all of them are of great value in enhancing the work of the body therapist. In my experience, it is best to stay with old favourites and 'keep it simple' when working with frail persons. One or two base oils have good therapeutic properties for the skin, such as almond and jojoba. When treating an older person, I have found that one drop of essential oil is enough when blended with the base oil. In some cases I have only used half a drop of essential oil, just enough for the client to enjoy the familiar smell, without feeling overpowered by the fragrance. If the client has a chronic skin problem, I may only use base oil until the problem has improved, and then I may introduce an essential oil that the client can cope with. If the client is on a medicated cream for chronic skin conditions, I will not use essential oils. Always work with caution when using essential oils on the frail. Frail older people can have a skin reaction to some strong odours such as lavender, mint, sandalwood and tea-tree. Most plants from the mint family can be too strong for frail persons.

The following are a few of my favourite oils that I have found to be helpful and safe to use on the majority of my clients. I continue to use them.

Almond (Prunis amygdalus or Amygdalus communis)

This is my favourite base oil, as it has wonderful properties nutritionally, and it is beneficial for the skin. I have found that clients who have allergies to nuts, can cope with a mild application of almond oil. In the latter years I mainly use almond oil for facials, fingernail care, massage and reflexology. The oil is good for all skin types and helps relieve itching, soreness, dryness and inflammation. Calendula oil mixed with almond is very good for inflammation. Almond oil contains glucosides, minerals and vitamins. Rich in protein, it comes from the kernel of the nut.

Avocado pear oil (Persea americana)

Avocado oil is good for most skins, especially for dry and dehydrated skins, and it is helpful for treating psoriasis and eczema.

Jojoba oil (Simmondsia chinensis)

Jojoba oil is very good for inflamed skins, psoriasis, eczema, acne, hair care and for all skin types. I add a few drops with most essential oil treatments.

Carrot oil (Daucus carota)

Carrot oil is very good to add in an oil mixture or with base oil for facials and fingernail care. It is also good for relieving itching, dryness, mild psoriasis and eczema.

Lavender (Lavandula angustifolia)

I use lavender oil for fingernail and toenail treatments and for a foot massage or foot spa. It is good for calming, relieving muscle pain and helps to stimulate blood flow. The oils have antiseptic and antibacterial properties. Lavender can be too strong for some frail persons and some people can have an allergy to lavender, so use with caution.

Marigold (Calendula officinalis)

I use calendula oil in all my treatments as I have found it to be very good to use direct on to the skin to soothe inflammation, especially after waxing or eyebrow shaping. Many of my older clients have found the oil can provide instant relief after hair removal. Calendula oil is also used in fingernail oil treatments, and added to cosmetic creams for skin care treatments. The oil is good for wound healing, acne, boils, tinea, bites and stings, inflammation, and even for varicose veins. It has antiseptic, detoxifying and anti-inflammatory properties.

Chamomile (Chamomilla matricaria)

Chamomile oil is added to most oil bases as it has antiallergenic and carminative properties. Chamomile oil is soothing and induces relaxation in a massage.

Tea-tree (Melaleuca alternifolia)

Tea-tree has the tendency to irritate the skin if applied directly without base oil. It can be too strong to use on a frail person in a massage. I mainly use tea-tree for its anti-inflammatory and antifungal properties that are used as a cleanser and added to fingernail oil treatment. Tea-tree oil can be overpowering to the senses and it would probably be best to use a tiny drop of oil diluted either in water or base oil. The oil is also useful for ringworm and fungi, cold sores, and for mild acne. It has proved very satisfactory in healing wounds.

Neroli (Citrus aurantium)

Neroli oil has a sweet 'orange blossom' scent and it is calming to the senses. I use a drop of this oil in face massage and reflexology. Many of my older clients enjoy the fragrance of this oil and comment that it reminds them of a perfume they used to wear when they were younger. This oil can help the client to relax with its calming properties.

Lemon (Citrus limon)

I mainly use lemon oil in a fingernail oil mixture. The smell of lemon oil can be too strong for some frail people.

ESSENTIAL OIL RECIPES

Fingernail essential oil treatment for older persons to help combat infections

Into a 10ml bottle (2 tablespoons), add:

> 9ml almond oil
>
> 1½ drops of jojoba oil
>
> ½ drop lavender oil (omit if allergic)
>
> ½ drop lemon oil
>
> ½ drop tea-tree oil
>
> 1 drop carrot oil
>
> 1 drop calendula oil.

Special fingernail base oil treatment for very frail persons unable to use scented oils

Into a 5ml bottle (1 tablespoon), add:

> 4ml almond oil
>
> 1 drop carrot oil
>
> 1 drop calendula oil.

This mixture will benefit the client's skin and help nourish the fingernails. Essential oils have a natural affinity with the body's own natural oils. This is why the nails look good after fingernail oil treatment, and the skin will look good after body therapy treatment. The essential oil recipes can also be used for removing stubborn dirt and faecal matter underneath the free-edge of the fingernails. It also helps to soften hard cuticles.

Herbal medicine

Herbal preparations have great value when used in a programme of 'self-care preventive medicine'. Some herbs are noted for their delightful culinary flavours that work gently on the digestive system. For example, as a good mouth wash for a sore throat, or for mouth and gum problems, and to help combat bad breath, a mixed herbal infusion of calendula and thyme will be helpful if gargled. Marigold infusion helps with calming inflammation. Lemon balm is a wonderful relaxant tea to have first thing in the morning; it relieves discomfort in the digestive system.

I use herbs as an infusion for external use in therapy treatments. A herbal infusion can be used as a facial skin freshener and cotton pads can be soaked in an infusion and used as eye pads to help soothe sore and tired eyes. Herbal infusions are also good for soaking feet and hands.

My four favourite herbal infusions are:

LAVENDER (LAVANDULA ANGUSTIFOLIA)

Wonderful for soaking feet and the hands. Has antibacterial properties.

MARIGOLD (CALENDULA OFFICINALIS)

Great for most treatments, mainly to help soothe inflammation.

I use a calendula infusion after waxing the face as it soothes the redness of the skin and helps it to fade quickly. Calendula is good for all skin problems.

ALOE (ALOE VERA)

The gel from the aloe plant can help to soothe inflamed skin, especially after a waxing procedure. Aloe gel or calendula oil helps to relieve the sting or pain when removing unwanted hair. I found the gel to be very good for waxing procedures and eyebrow shaping, and soothing for burns.

CHAMOMILE (CHAMOMILLA MATRICARIA)
Use as a face freshener and to help soothe tired or sore eyes.

Clients benefit greatly from these herbal infusions as they are soothing and gentle and they do not seem to cause irritation to the skin of older clients. The infusions I make up are more diluted to suit an older frail person.

Making an infusion for older or frail people

½ tsp dried herb to cup or 1½ cups of warm water

or

1½ tsp fresh herbs to cup or 1½ cups of warm water.

Infusions have a short life (about 2–4 days) and should be stored in a cool place. Once an infusion becomes rancid, it must be disposed of immediately. I find it best to make up herbal infusions each day.

CREATIVE VISUALISATION

Creative visualisation is a technique that uses the mind's ability to imagine sights, sounds, movements and other sensory experiences as a means of inducing specific physical reactions in the body, or to encourage changes in a client's emotional outlook. For example, the practitioner can focus on a particular body part that needs attention, and visualise that the body part is in its previous 'healthy' state. Although the physical part of the body will not be restored to its full natural health, the client may feel better coping with her illness over a period of time. Another way of using creative visualisation is to allow the client to reminisce about a place she has visited in the past that was pleasant, encouraging her to see, feel and enjoy the happiness of this special place. Creative visualisation works in many ways and is based on individual acceptance. The practitioner alone can use creative visualisation without a client's cooperation and maintain positive results. The same applies to colour therapy.

COLOUR THERAPY

Colour therapy works in a similar way to creative visualisation, except that specific colours are used for certain parts of the body, for certain illnesses, for different emotions, and/or spiritual development. Depending on how the practitioner was taught, she will use colour imagery for one of the above or more. Colour is very effective and can work strongly on our moods and emotions. The change of the seasons demonstrates how we may feel and how it can affect our moods. A dull, cold, overcast day can induce a depressed feeling, whereas in warm sunshine we can receive a feeling of vitality and golden warmth enlightening our spirit, thus creating more energy.

Creative visualisation and colour therapy work well in all body work treatment and with other therapies (Figure 6.4).

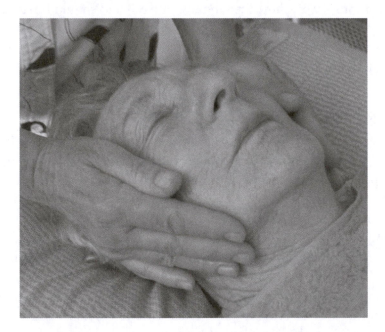

FIGURE 6.4 The client receives a facial massage followed by face reflexology. Creative visualisation and colour therapy can be used with these two body therapies.

CHAPTER 7

Reflexology and Face Reflexology for People in Care

WHAT IS REFLEXOLOGY?

The Reflexology Association of Australia (n.d.) says:

> Reflexology is based on the principle that all parts of the body are reflected on the feet, hands, face and ears. It is the application of pressure and soothing techniques to these parts of the body. Pressure points are also referred to as Reflex points. Reflexology is known as an holistic, non-invasive therapy, which complements other therapies and modern medicine.

Reflexology is an art, a science and a skill that uses gentle pressure and manipulation of the feet, hands, face and ears. Reflexologists believe that the foot, ear, face or hand mirrors the body (Figure 7.1). A compression technique is used on specific reflexes on the face, hands and feet that enables the organs and body parts to be re-energised and rebalanced.

Relaxation is the first step towards normalising nerve and blood supply to all areas of the body, thus encouraging better circulation for the supply of nutrients and oxygen to the cells. It then follows that glands are more able to normalise their function.

The inside edge of the foot resembles the spine and is the reflex point of the spine on the body. The head sits at its upper end (the big toe), the shoulders are located at the top of the ball of the foot. The waist is at the mid-line of the foot in its arch and the buttocks are the heel.

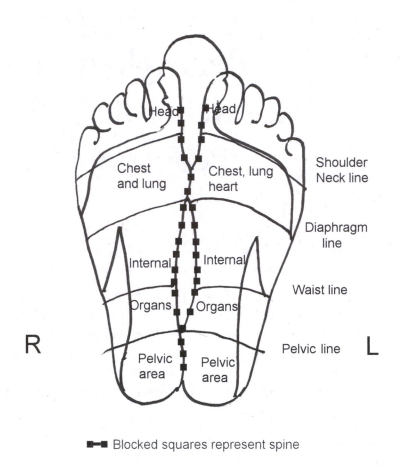

Blocked squares represent spine

FIGURE 7.1 The soles of the feet mirror the body.

Observing your own foot you will notice the similarity between its structure and the structure of your spine (Figure 7.2). The spine has 33 bones* and the sides of the feet have 26 bones in each foot. You may also notice that where your feet hurt, that is where your body is causing you concern at the same time. The little toe side is the lateral (outside) of the body, and the medial side is the centre of the body.

> * It was once thought that the spine had 26 bones, equal to the bones in the feet. This is because the sacral and coccyx bones are fused, therefore placing them as one for the sacral and one for the coccyx. The sacral bones consist of five fused bones and

the coccyx has four fused bones thus making 33 bones in the spine. Breaking the spine into segments, there are the cervicals (neck) 7, thoracic 12, lumbar 5, sacral 5 and the coccyx 4.

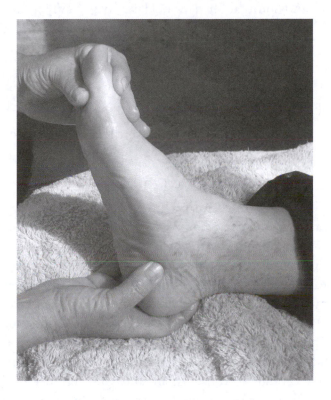

FIGURE 7.2 The reflex points for the spine are along the arch of the foot.

WHAT IS THE DIFFERENCE BETWEEN REFLEXOLOGY AND ACUPRESSURE?

Acupressure and reflexology are both bodywork techniques which involve applying pressure to specific points on the body for the purpose of addressing health complaints, but these techniques are very different. Acupressure involves points on the whole body, while reflexology concentrates on the reflex points on the feet, hands, face and ears which relate to the organs and glands of the body. Acupressure is based on the concept of *Chi* or *Qi*, defined in Traditional Chinese Medicine (TCM) as an essential life force that flows through the body circulating through invisible passageways residing in the body's interior (these are referred to as meridians).

The movement or flow of Chi is said to vary with the mental, physical and spiritual changes of daily living. When Chi flows evenly, harmony and good health are possible. If Chi circulation is stagnant, overstimulated or unbalanced, illness is likely.

On the skin there are specific places or points called acupoints where Chi may be accessed and guided by the practitioner using deep finger pressure.

On frail, sensitive skin, deep pressure should be avoided.

HOW DOES REFLEXOLOGY HELP?

Reflexology is non-intrusive, promotes relaxation, can help induce sleep, help nature achieve homeostasis and can improve blood and lymphatic circulation. Unblocking nerve impulses it can assist sciatic pain, relieve stress levels, reduce pain and constipation and headaches and promote elimination of toxins. It can help to improve muscle tension thereby improving the outlook on life. It is a very helpful therapy when used in conjunction with complementary therapies and conventional medicine.

Reflexology helps the body normalise by working through both the central nervous system and the peripheral nervous system. When pressure is applied through the skin of the feet both the spinal nerves and the sympathetic nerves of the blood vessels are affected. If an organ or gland is hyperactive then reflexology also works through the parasympathetic system during the relaxation process.

When an older person accepts this therapy, she can generally cope better and look forward to further treatments. Some frail persons may not fully understand the benefits of reflexology, but many enjoy the touch and the feeling of being cared for; the touch of a therapist brings them into a state of relaxation. With frail older people, the reflexologist may find that the client's best option of treatment may be on the hands or face. Some reasons are:

- the client is not very mobile in moving her feet into position

- the client has sore or infected feet

- the client has foot sores or injury

- the client may be suffering with circulation abnormalities

- the client has lost a limb/limbs

- the client does not like having her feet touched.

If the client is able to have foot reflexology, it is not always practical to give a foot bath to bed-confined clients. The best method is to give a 'towel clean' (the feet cleaned with a warm towel and cleanser). If treating the hands, soak the client's hands in a bowl or use the 'towel clean' method for hand reflexology.

The length of time spent working on a frail person will depend on how she is coping. The therapist will be able to assess the client's condition. I have found that 20 minutes is long enough for older people when working on their hands or face. For the feet, I have worked about 30 to 45 minutes, or less, depending on how the client is feeling on the day of treatment.

Working over the hand reflexes can be very challenging for the therapist as some older clients are so glad to have someone touch their hands that they will often grab the therapist's hand and not let go. This can make it difficult to work over the client's reflex/ pressure points. The best way I have found to cope with this problem is to gently massage the hand; this often helps the client to relax. If the client is not relaxed, I simply continue with gently massaging the hand and slowly introduce some slight pressure to the points over the hand, similar to the method I use for face reflexology. This technique can be as beneficial to the client as if I was giving her a full hand reflexology session.

Difficulties can also apply to the feet. Clients who are not used to touch, or do not understand instructions, can tighten their muscles by stretching out their feet or pulling them towards their abdomen in a foetal position. This is common with clients who suffer some form of dementia. Reflexology foot relaxing massage may help to relax the client. I have found that some clients with dementia will have difficulty in cooperating and will persist in moving their feet all through the session. In such circumstances, it is best to abort working on the feet and try the hands or face. Always work out what is best for the client.

Treating older and frail people can be challenging for the therapist and it is preferable that the therapist remains flexible and able to improvise; this may involve a change in their approach and ideas, very different from treating clients in a salon or clinic.

Many older persons can enjoy reflexology to the hands, face or feet with positive benefits, especially for those with dementia, as reflexology can induce relaxation and calmness (Figure 7.3). After the session, clients can remain relaxed and happy for the rest of the day. In many cases, a reflexology treatment has helped clients who suffer with constipation by making them relax, thus assisting with elimination from the colon.

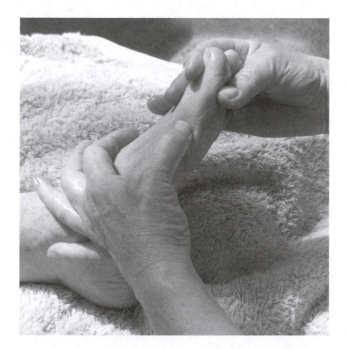

FIGURE 7.3 The reflex points for the cervicals are on the medial side of the foot near the base of the big toe.

FACE REFLEXOLOGY

Face reflexology is as old as feet and hand reflexology, though there has not been a lot of information on this topic until recently. There are now a few textbooks that incorporate face reflexology into other body therapies. It is difficult to pin-point all the reflex and pressure points and there are many areas in which the practitioner can advance their knowledge and techniques by keeping abreast of current developments. Each practitioner who tutors in this topic may vary from another tutor and all are equally correct. For the student this can be confusing. The best method is to work with intuition, allowing yourself to explore the possibilities of forming your own ideas as to how to find and work the reflex or pressure points. Feedback from clients and friends is essential and it is the main factor that can help a student to remain focused while getting started.

When I had completed my massage and reflexology certificate courses, I soon became aware of the reflexology and pressure points, especially when I was giving a client a facial. It was during my studies in naturopathy that I discovered a book published in the 1970s by Viktoras Kulvinskas, *Survival in the 21st Century* (1975); it contained a chapter on reflexology. In this chapter I found an illustration of a face showing reflex points and a few acupressure points. I was astounded to find the points indicated on this drawing were the same, or similar, to the points I had been working on previously with my clients during their facials. In this case 'intuition' had paid off. I continue to use the Viktoras chart and I have become very familiar with many of its reflex points, working to a particular method, elements of which I have incorporated into this chapter. Over the years I have found these techniques satisfactory. The feedback from clients has been useful and encouraging.

HOW DOES FACE REFLEXOLOGY WORK?

Face reflexology incorporates techniques that stimulate the reflexes of the head, forehead, face, jaw, ears, throat and the sides of the neck. It improves blood circulation and energy flow; it also helps release tension, improves skin texture, helps disperse impurities deep within the pores of the skin, helps relieve the perils of minor skin conditions and aids in lymphatic drainage. Regular treatments tend to firm the muscles of the face and jaw, providing a natural, non-surgical facelift. Face reflexology can be used in conjunction with ear reflexology, facials, massage, face acupressure, aromatherapy, colour therapy and Traditional Chinese Medicine face mapping.

Face reflexology gently decreases blockages, restores balances within the body system and lowers stress levels. Face reflexology should be worked at a slower pace than when working on the feet. This is because the head, face and neck are delicate areas and should be treated with caution.

The method for applying face reflexology is to work over the face with fingers and thumb, but in a different way from the technique used on the feet and hands. The method used over the feet and hands is to use the fingers and thumb in a 'caterpillar'-like movement. Working the reflex and pressure points over the face and neck involves light pressure to the points. The fingers are held on the reflex or pressure point for a few seconds or longer if there are indications of congestion such as hard bumps, granules like crystals, depressions in the skin or build-up of fluid. More than one reflex point can be done at the same time, for example, the kidney and adrenals and the liver and spleen reflex points. Pressure should be firm but not uncomfortable for the client. Some clients may not be able to cope with too much pressure. Hold the pressure, then release, and apply again. Each point is worked over three times. Work carefully and assess the client as you progress through the treatment. Look for signals from the client that the pressure is too hard or that she has had enough. This can be indicated by the client:

- moving her head
- twitching her face and pulling facial expressions
- touching her face
- scratching.

This is most important if the client is not able to communicate. Most clients can tell you what they are experiencing. Always finish the treatment with soft flowing massage movements.

Before commencement of face reflexology, the face should be cleansed and this followed by a gentle massage. Massage helps to relax the client's face muscles and prepare her for the treatment.

CONTRAINDICATIONS

Face reflexology can be applied safely without causing harm to the client providing care is taken when working on the head, around the neck and over the face. However, there are a few exceptions when face reflexology would not be appropriate, or should be used with caution. Examples are:

- over new scars or burns

- where there are skin infections

- if there is a discharge from any part of the face

- where there are other visible inflammatory lesions

- if the client is unable to cope with touch

- if the client has a neck disorder

- if the client is having chemotherapy or radiation therapy

- if the client has a cold or a flu virus (even if she is getting over the illness)

- if the client has a recent head injury

- if there are uncontrollable movements of the head and face

- if the client experiences high or low blood pressure

- if the client has recently taken alcoholic beverages

- if the client is on sedative medication

- if the client is unable to cooperate.

Clients with a sensitive skin should not be worked on any longer than 10–15 minutes or even less, depending on the severity of the skin condition. Always use light pressure on sensitive skins and clients with poor skin conditions.

FACE REFLEXOLOGY FOR OLDER PEOPLE

Face reflexology (sometimes referred to as facial reflexology) is one of the most frequently used therapies that I have found to be beneficial to many of my older clients and for those in palliative care. It is one therapy I have found to be safe and which can be applied to sensitive skin without harmful side effects. Many of my older clients have remarked how much they enjoy this therapy and continue to have it as their regular treatment. I also incorporate this therapy into a facial treatment.

FACE REFLEXOLOGY POINTS AND HEAD ANATOMY

While working and concentrating on the face and head reflexes, the student needs at the same time to be aware that the brain, face nerves, face muscles, face skeletal bones, the sensory organs and circulatory systems are also being incorporated into the treatment. It is important for the student to have an understanding of face anatomy as well as full body anatomy and physiology functions. I do not intend to teach the reader the foundations of anatomy and physiology as each student and practitioner should be well informed in this subject before venturing into this modality or any other body therapy.

A little more emphasis should be placed on the digestive system, in that it is the key organ distributing nutrients into the cells of the body, nourishing organs and glands, and helping maintain their functions; the digestive system reacts instantly to the stimulation on the reflex points.

I have found that working on the digestive reflexes will often stimulate the gastric juices in the stomach and help with elimination, much to the satisfaction (or embarrassment) of many clients.

1. Head relaxer
2. Pituitary
3. Pineal
4. Sinuses
5. Eyes (reflex points for kidneys/adrenals)
6. Stomach and for constipation
7. Bladder
8. Reflex point for leg cramp

9. Stomach
10. Mouth, teeth and gums
11. Lymphatic drainage
12. Top helix of ear
13. Outer ear
14. Lobule of ear
15. Tragus of ear

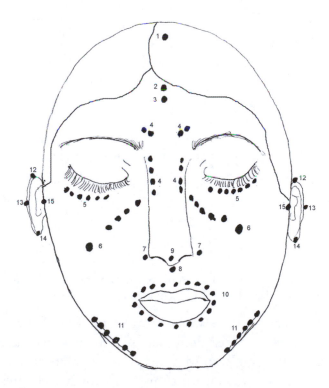

The skull can be worked over with gentle pressure, helping to relieve head tension and stress and improve circulation.

FIGURE 7.4 This face chart shows the additional reflex points I incorporate into my face therapy.

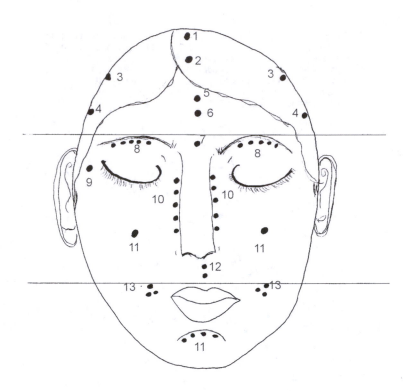

1. Brain stimulation
2. Reproductive organs
3. Memory
4. Sciatica
5. Sympathetic nerve
6. Mentality/pelvic region
7. Headache

8. Digestion
9. Liver
10. Intestines
11. Constipation
12. Spleen and pancreas
13. Lungs

FIGURE 7.5 This face chart shows some of the reflex points, taken from Viktoras' illustrated face chart, that I include in my face reflexology.

Some additional points relate to areas of the face that are not actually pressure or reflex points, as seen in the face chart in Figure 7.4. For example, in working pressure points around the mouth, you are also working the gums, teeth, tongue. For pressure points relating to kidneys/adrenals, you are working around the eyes. The face chart in Figure 7.5 shows some valid reflex points from Viktoras Kulvinskas' face drawing used in conjunction with the points on Figure 7.4.

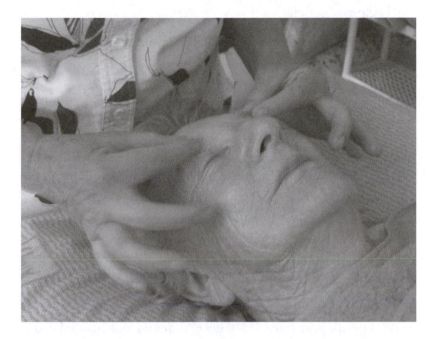

FIGURE 7.6 Along the eyebrow line are reflex points for digestion.

The face is divided into three sections

1. Top region (largest part): top of head and forehead.

2. Middle region: between eyebrows and top upper lip.

3. Lower region (smallest part): from top lip down through the chin and neck.

Top region

THE SKULL

Top part of the head. Frontal and occipital bone and frontalis and occipitals muscles.

1. Centre of skull: reflex point to stimulate body and centre of spine and centre for brain stimulation.

2. From centre of head to sides of head: stimulation for reproductive organs, internal organs and brain. Stimulate blood flow and oil flow.

3. Back of head: stimulation of brain, nerves, helps blood flow, helps relieve head tension and induce relaxation. May help shed dead skin cells and increase oil flow in the hair.

BASE OF THE SKULL

Occipital bone and occipitalis muscle.

1. Centre base of occipital bone, near cervicals: releases tension in head, jaw, may stimulate saliva. Reflex point for cervicals and spine. May help migraine and headache and relieve head tension.

THE FOREHEAD

Frontal bone and frontalis muscle.

1. Centre top towards hair line: pituitary and pineal glands. Nerve and mental stimulation.

2. Middle centre, above eyebrows: frontal sinuses, mentality.

3. Centre of brows: reflex point for headache, ethmoid sinuses and bladder.

SIDE OF HEAD

Frontal, temporal and parietal bones. Frontalis, temporalis and occipitalis muscles.

1. From centre of hairline down to top side: memory (1 o'clock), sciatica (2 o'clock), reproductive organs just behind these two reflex points towards centre skull.

2. 4 o'clock close to temporal bone: headache.

Middle region

EYEBROW LINE

Frontal, occipital and sphenoid bones. Frontalis, corrugator supercilii muscles.

1. In between brows: ethmoid sinuses. May help relieve headache.

2. Underneath the brow line and above eye socket: helpful towards digestion and stomach disorders.

THE EYES

Sphenoid, ethmoid and lacrimal bones. Orbicularis oculi muscle, levator palpebrae superioris muscles under eyes and cheeks.

RIGHT EYE

1. Outer corner of eye: liver and gall bladder.

2. Underneath eye close to lower lash line: kidney and adrenals.

LEFT EYE

1. Outer corner of eye: spleen, heart and for wind problems.

2. Underneath eye close to lower lash line: kidney and adrenals.

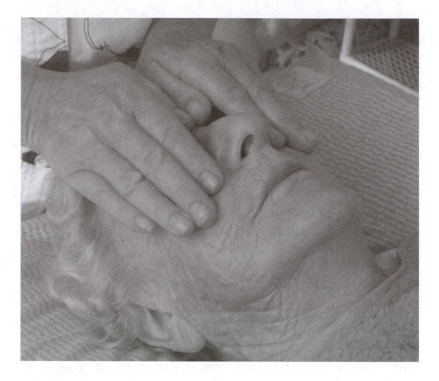

FIGURE 7.7 Cupping the eyes is soothing and relaxing for the client.

Cheeks

Zygomatic bones. Buccinator, zygomaticus major muscle.

Right cheek

1. Middle of cheek in line with pupil: maxillas sinuses, digestion and for constipation.

2. Inner cheek bone close to nostril: bladder, sinuses, top right gum.

Left cheek

1. Middle of cheek in line with pupil: sinuses and digestion.

2. Inner cheek bone close to nostril: bladder, sinuses, top left gum.

3. Over cheek bone: helps to relieve facial pain.

THE NOSE

Nasal, frontal and palatine bones. Nasal cartilage.

1. Across the nose and sides of the nose: sinuses, helps relieve nose blockage and allergies.

2. From the bridge of nose down the sides of nose to nostrils: for the intestines.

3. Tip of nose: stomach.

4. Underneath nose, centre of upper top lip: leg muscle cramps.

Lower region

UPPER TOP LIP AND MOUTH

Mandible, zygomatic and maxilla bones. Orbicularis oris, sides of mouth. Levator labii superioris, buccinator, risorius, masseter, temporalis muscles.

1. Join to septum of nose: leg muscle cramp.

2. Centre of upper lip: pancreas and spleen.

MOUTH

1. Corner of mouth left and right: lungs. Stimulate salivary glands. Bottom gums, teeth, tongue.

CHIN

Mandible bone. Mentalis, buccinator muscles.

1. Centre of chin: heart.

2. In crease of chin: for constipation.

The above will also act as reflex points for bottom gums, teeth and tongue.

NECK

Cervical bones and hyoid bone. Platysma and sternocleidomastoid muscles.

1. Front, centre of neck: thyroid and parathyroid. Sore throat. Reflex points for oesophagus and trachea.

2. Back, 7th cervical: cervicals, spine, muscle tension, stiff and sore neck.

The ears

While massaging the sides of the face I gently work around the ears using pressure behind the ears and in front of the head flap of the ear (tragus). I hold the wide ridge (superior part of the ear: reflex points for foot, leg, knee, hip, lower spine) and the bottom lobe of the ear at the same time for the brain, jaw, head (inferior section). I then change position, to holding the lateral and medial side of the ear. The lateral side-long groove (scaphoid fossa: reflex points for hand, wrist, elbow, arm and shoulder) is very good for blood circulation. The medial side, over the tragus, is the adrenal point. When finished, I cup my hands over the ear and this helps towards soothing sore ears and loosens ear wax.

> Holding the pressure points around the ears helps to unblock ears when travelling on a plane. If the client is wearing a hearing aid, do not work near the ears (Figure 7.8). Gentle cupping may be alright.

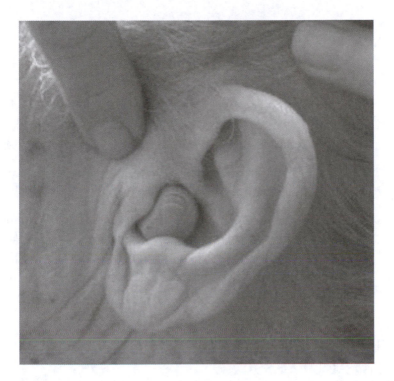

FIGURE 7.8 Care must be taken when treating a client around the ears if the client is wearing a hearing aid.

FACE REFLEXOLOGY FOR FRAIL PERSONS

Face reflexology is beneficial for elderly clients and those with a disability. Clients can be worked on either in a sitting or lying position, though a lying position is more practical, as the client can be more relaxed without having to use her muscles to support a sitting position. The following list shows some of the benefits a client receives from a face reflexology session.

- The lines of the face become relaxed.

- The client benefits from toxins eliminating from the skin.

- The client's skin is refreshed, smooth and cleaned.

- The therapy does not aggravate the skin.

- The client is very relaxed throughout and after a session.

- Minor skin problems are minimised either through or after a session.

- Aromatherapy oils with face reflexology help relax the client and work in removing dirt particles from the skin and rejuvenating the skin pores.

- Headache, sinus problems, earache and muscle tension, including leg cramps, may be relieved.

Clients with severe skin conditions may require only a gentle pressure of light effleurage movement by contouring the face for a few minutes or less, depending how poor, or sore, the skin may look. Light touch is essential when working on frail, sensitive skin.

CHINESE FACE READING AND ACUPRESSURE

Chinese face reading is a tradition that reaches back thousands of years, probably originating around the sixth century BC. It is based on the theory that the face broadcasts a person's energetic profile as well as aspects of character and personality. The Chinese art of face reading is a very involved system that classifies facial features by colour of the skin, texture of the skin, shape of face, skin eruptions, lines and disfigurements.

The origins of acupressure are as ancient as the instinctive impulse to hold your forehead or temples when you have a headache. Everyone at one time or another has used his or her hands spontaneously to hold tense or painful places of the body. More than 5000 years ago, the Chinese discovered that pressing certain points on the body relieved pain where it occurred and also benefited other parts of the body more remote from the pain and pressure point. Gradually they discovered other locations that not only alleviated pain but influenced the functioning of certain internal organs.

As a beauty therapist I have found Chinese face reading very helpful when diagnosing skin problems and why they may have occurred. The most common skin ailment that many people may suffer from sometime in their life is acne. In Chinese face reading acne on the *forehead and temples* may indicate digestive disorders such as difficulty breaking down certain foods. It could also relate to a toxin build-up of hair products, (shampoos, dyes), wearing dirty caps or hats and a build-up of using contaminated cosmetics. Acne on the *cheeks* may be caused through stress, stomach problems, too much sugar, dirty mobile phones, dirty pillow cases and use of dirty cosmetic accessories (i.e. cosmetic brushes). The *nose* displaying acne indicates poor diet and gastrointestinal disturbances.

The different colour hues of the skin can also give a therapist an indication of what may be happening internally. For example if a person has a *ruddy hue* (red) they may have either high blood pressure, heart or circulatory imbalance, hormonal changes in menopause, dehydration or skin sensitivity. A *pink flushed* skin can also relate to sensitivity, heat, hormonal disturbance, illness, fever, and certain medications, or the client may have just completed some physical activity such as exercise or running. A *yellow or brown* undertone may relate to liver or kidney imbalance, illness or fever. A *greenish* tone may be due to a gall bladder imbalance, fever, influenza, overload of alcohol, drugs, fatty foods or contaminated foods. A *blue hue* around the eyes may indicate a sluggish digestive system or overtiredness. If there is blue around the lips this may indicate a heart or circulatory imbalance.

Face reflexology is a recent development in Australia and there are several differing face charts in textbooks and on the internet. In common are particular points that relate to the organs and glands of the body. This can be confusing to the student. Unlike foot reflexology, face reflexology can be taught by the tutor using their experience and knowledge to guide the student to using a specific face map chart. With experience a practitioner can begin incorporating their own findings and experiment with various facial points using client feedback. The 'positive' client feedback provides the evidence to support face reflexology therapeutic claims.

Face massage before and after applying face reflexology aids circulation, improves skin tone by releasing impurities from the pores of the skin and also assists in toning face muscles.

CONCLUSION

In my experience, using Viktoras' face reflexology points, and developing a few of my own methods, works well with frail clients, especially when I am unable to work on the feet or hands. Face reflexology and reflexology in general is widely accepted in my professional work and I hope to see that it is used as one of the mainstream therapies in the near future, especially in aged care and palliative care. It would be a lucrative business market, in addition to promoting good health.

CHAPTER 8

Home Visits and Hospital Visits

HOME VISITS

Home visits involve running a mobile service to a client's private residence. Home visits can be available to clients of all age groups whether they are in good health or ill health. Beauty therapists and hairdressers make regular home visits for wedding makeovers, for mothers in post-natal care, and for clients who are unable to visit a salon. The therapist can cater for most beauty therapy treatments. The demand for home visits for beauty therapy, hairdressing and for natural therapy treatments has increased in the last decade and will probably continue to grow due to older people remaining in their homes longer. The focus in this chapter is mainly on frail and older persons.

VISITING A CLIENT

When a person is making an appointment the therapist should make sure she gets all the details before making a commitment, otherwise she may find she has gone on a 'bogus' call. If the client is known to the therapist, this is not a problem. The following questions may be a helpful guide:

- Seek name, address, phone contact number.

- Ask for specific directions of how to get there, even if you do know how, this gives a clear indication that the caller is making a genuine appointment.

- Discuss payment details.

- Mention any other requests or concerns before finalising the appointment.

If the appointment has been made a few days or weeks in advance, always phone the client the day before to make sure she still wants the appointment. If she does, give her an estimated time of arrival.

> Older people sometimes forget an appointment or become ill, so it is always best to phone ahead before visiting.

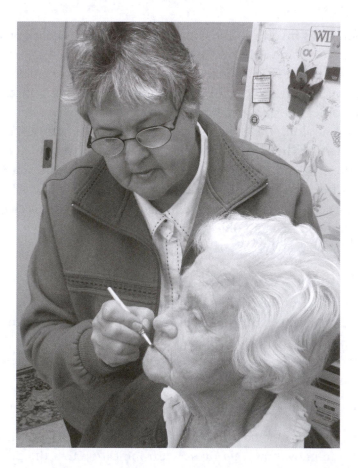

FIGURE 8.1 The therapist visits an elderly woman aged 101. The client enjoys having regular treatments finishing with a light makeup.

Day of client's appointment

The first contact with a client may be in her home and the therapist will need to familiarise herself with the setting of the room and know where best to give the client her treatment. Try to make an area safe and suitable for work and comfortable for the client. Assess the client's capability. Sometimes when a client is making an appointment, she can sound very able, which can give the impression that she has good mobility. This may not be the case when the therapist has completed the client's assessment. The reverse can also be true; a person may give details of her poor mobility, but the therapist may find that she is quite capable of movement during treatment.

CONTRACTS AND AGREEMENT FORMS

A contract or agreement form consists of specific agreements made between the therapist and the client. The client agrees to the therapist (and perhaps an assistant) visiting her at home to give her therapy treatment. An agreement form can also specify payment conditions that the therapist may claim should a client forget or refuse to have treatment, once the therapist has arrived at the client's home. Although agreement forms are not compulsory, they are an asset to cover any 'misunderstandings' that may occur between the therapist and the client. Fortunately, I seldom use them, but I do see it could be an issue in the future with the ever-changing rules regarding insurance policies and government regulations for practitioners working with people in care.

Client contract for home visits

Before commencing treatment, the therapist may ask the client to sign a contract. If the client wants to continue with her treatments, the contract is valid until the client discontinues treatment. The following contract is a guide the therapist may like to follow or, alternatively, she can make up her own contract, should it be necessary.

AGREEMENT FORM

Between _____ (the therapist)

and _____ (the client)

of _____ (street, town)

The therapist agrees to provide the selected services including

_____

(state the treatments) on the following terms:

1. The client agrees that the therapist and her assistant may enter the client's premises to give treatment.

2. The client agrees to obtain the advice and consent of her medical practitioner for the treatment prior to commencement if that is necessary.

3. The client agrees to advise the therapist of any relevant medical information which may be contraindicated to the treatment.

4. The client agrees that the therapist will not undertake any lifting, domestic assistance or nursing care.

5. The client agrees to supply her own clean linen (for hygiene reasons).

6. The client agrees that there will be no unreasonable interruptions during treatment, such as taking phone calls for long conversations, having visitors interrupt, wasting the therapist's time.

7. The client agrees to pay the therapist's specified costs at the time of consultation.

8. The client may cancel the agreement for services, but if notice of the cancellation is not given in reasonable time, the client agrees she will be liable for any travel expenses arising from the failure to cancel.

9. The client will nominate a relative or friend who will be responsible for expenses if the client is unable to make transactions or appointments.

10. The client agrees not to smoke prior to or during the treatment.

Signed _____

dated _____ (client)

Signed _____

dated _____ (therapist)

Signed _____

dated _____ (assistant)

GUIDANCE NOTES

The following notes relate to points 4, 6, 9 and 10 in the contract:

4. Many elderly people live on their own, and become reliant on carers and relatives to do their odd jobs and general house cleaning. Some older persons can be very lonely and sometimes try to make the therapist's visit last longer.

   Delaying tactics include:

   - taking their time to get ready for the treatment

   - offering cups of tea

   - finding some way to keep the therapist's attention.

   They will ask the therapist to do things and possibly to run errands. As a professional, the therapist must make it clear that she is there to give treatment. This may sound harsh but, if rules are not made clear, the therapist may find that she has been coaxed into being the 'errand' girl, and it will probably always be expected each time the therapist visits. However, on some occasions I have stopped to share a cup of tea when I have had extra time to spare. This has only happened with clients who have been on my appointment books for a long time.

6. It can be difficult for the therapist if the client has a lot of interruptions while she is trying to give her client treatment. The client will benefit from her treatment in a quiet environment.

9. A relative or close friend must be responsible for the client's expenses if the client is unable to communicate, deal with money transactions or make appointments.

10. This is optional, and it is between the therapist and client. However, it is best if neither the therapist nor the client smoke during the client's treatment.

On some occasions I have had to give a relative a contract to sign on behalf of a client in a nursing home. Some relatives who are in charge of the client's expenses will not always agree to the client having treatment, and the therapist could end up out of pocket if they go ahead, even on the client's wishes. Sadly, some relatives do not like to spend money on their family member as they do not see certain therapies being beneficial to the client, or their financial circumstances have changed.

Client contract for nursing home residents

The contract is similar to the home visit, but with fewer clauses. A 'trustee' may be the nursing staff or a guardian, as the client may have no relative in charge of expenses. Fortunately I have not used many contracts in nursing homes, although they could be a priority in the near future.

Readers have permission to download the following template from www.singingdragon.com/catalogue/9781848191785/resources for personal use with this programme.

AGREEMENT FORM

The therapist agrees to provide services of

_____

(state the treatments) on the following basis:

1. The client/relative/trustee agrees to the advice and consent of the doctor/nurse in charge to the treatment prior to commencement if that is necessary.

2. The client/relative/trustee agrees to advise the therapist of any relevant medical information which may be contraindicated to treatment.

3. The client/relative/trustee agrees that the therapist will not undertake any lifting, domestic assistance or nursing care.

4. The client/relative/trustee will arrange to pay for treatment at the time of each visit.

5. The client/relative/trustee may cancel this agreement at any time with notice before the next visit. Expenses may be incurred if the therapist is not notified prior to the visit.

I _____ (client/relative/trustee) give consent for _____ (name of client) of _____ (nursing home) to have _____ (specify treatment) on a weekly/ fortnightly/monthly basis.

Signed _____

dated _____ (client/relative/trustee)

THE CLIENT AT HOME
Setting up a safe and clean area

Visiting a client's home can be very challenging with regard to her living conditions. Some people live in small apartments, flats or units while others still remain in the family home. Some older clients that I have visited live alone while some have shared with a family member. Some younger people are cared for by their parents or by a relative, and share the facilities of the home. In most homes I have visited I have found that the client will often have a place ready for me to work. I always made sure the area was suitable for me to work in and if not, I would ask the client if I could use another area. Most people are happy to oblige. The therapist must think first of her own safety. Never work in conditions that can cause any difficulty in giving treatment to a client in their home.

This could arise due to:

- hygiene concerns

- safety issues (equipment and furniture, little room to manoeuvre)

- strain on the therapist's back (bending and stooping over chairs and low beds)

- interruptions (visitors, phone calls)

- uncontrollable animals (jumping up on the therapist)

- exposure to chemicals, tobacco smoke or other harmful products.

Interruptions

Unfortunately interruptions do happen during a treatment that may or may not be the fault of the client. The most annoying is the phone, when the client spends a lot of time talking to callers. To overcome this problem, the therapist should tell the client that her valuable time is costing money and that she has only so much time left for the session. Clients soon learn to be brief. It may sound mean, but if time-wasting is accepted, the therapist could end up being late for other appointments. This also applies to any other interruptions, such as visitors who intrude and take over the conversation. Sometimes it can be fine, if the client needs the support of a friend or relative to help in communication or if she is happier with company while she is having her treatment. This may be acceptable for some hair and beauty therapy treatments, but not for body work such as massage and reflexology, where it is preferable for the client to have a quiet atmosphere, isolated from others. Interruptions can also arise from regular callers such as volunteers from Meals on Wheels, district nurses, domestic carers and delivery merchants. If the therapist establishes regular appointments with the client, the client will be able to organise suitable times for her callers and this can prevent interruptions when the client is having treatment.

Living conditions

Visiting older people in their homes can be very special as they are always pleased to see a visitor. Older persons who live on their own can sometimes be very lonely and long for company. I have visited a few clients who had treatment mainly for my company and conversation (Figure 8.2). Some older people have very few visitors because members of their family may live in another town or country or maybe they have no family. If their mobility is not good and they are unable to get out on their own, they may rely on visitors to run their errands. This is one scenario. There are many more. Sometimes a person's living conditions can be very sparse with a few material comforts compared to those who are better off.

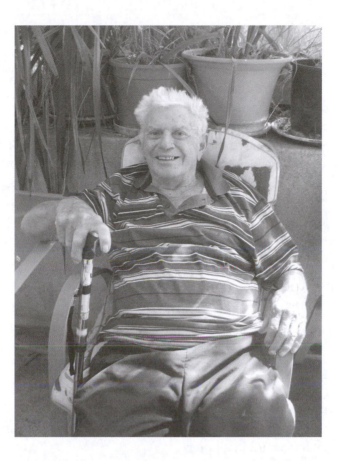

FIGURE 8.2 Male clients enjoy having treatments at home from a visiting therapist. The client has limited mobility and relies on a walking stick.

Animals often play an important role in companionship for an older person living alone. I have noticed that clients who have an animal friend to share their home are less stressed. The animals are just as pleased to see visitors as their owners, and they will greet a visitor at the door with a friendly woof or purr. Being an animal lover, I must confess I enjoy my visits where there is a resident 'furry' friend as they make a great conversation topic. Many an animal will curl up beside their owner while she is having her treatment. This creates a very 'relaxed' atmosphere for both the therapist and the client.

In my early days as a novice therapist I made regular fortnightly visits to an older woman. She had a beautiful white and black cat named Missy. When I had completed my client's massage, Missy would jump up on a footstool for me to give her a massage. She would purr in ecstasy, turning and tossing to the sheer joy of every stroke. This became a regular routine with Missy until she had an accident and was hit by a car. While her leg was mending she was unable to climb on to stools or chairs and soon gave up trying. Once the fracture was mended, she had lost interest in having a massage due to the stiffness in her leg and I was unable to get down on the floor level due to pain and swelling in my knees.

VISITING A CLIENT IN HOSPITAL

An appointment is often made by the client or sometimes by the hospital staff. When visiting a client in the hospital always check with nursing staff first to ensure that:

- the client is free to take visitors

- the equipment the therapist will use is approved. Some machinery can interfere with hospital equipment, this includes mobile phones

- the client is permitted to have the treatment she has asked for (e.g. facial waxing post-surgery)

- staff assistance is available if required or for any items that may be needed such as clean towels.

It is not a good idea to give a client a wax treatment on the day of their surgical operation, especially an older client. Their immunity may be lowered and they can easily pick up an infection, especially if there is the slightest skin nick or bleeding after waxing. Pathogens spread quickly when a person's immunity is low. It is best to leave any removal of unwanted hair until the client has recovered from their operation. Nail varnish should not be applied to the fingernails or toenails before a client undergoes any surgical procedures due to diagnostic requirements.

When the client's assessment is completed, the therapist may set up the equipment or cosmetics, placing them on the hospital mobile bed tray/table. Make sure the client has privacy by pulling a curtain around her bed if she is sharing a room. If the client is in a single room, close the door and place a Do Not Disturb sign outside the door.

PALLIATIVE CARE CLIENTS

The therapist may be asked to go on a hospital visit or house call to a client who has a long-term illness. She may be in the last days of her illness. In these cases, most clients will probably only want a short service, like a massage or reflexology or a service mainly to tidy up and help them feel better, freed from annoying problems such as unwanted facial hair or broken fingernails. Depending on illness or reaction to medication, the latter two beauty services are the most sought after. Some clients prefer to have a massage or reflexology treatment as the two favoured body therapies. Clients who are dealing with a long-term illness will probably be in pain or may have difficulty in holding a comfortable position for long periods of time. The therapist may need to work quickly and carefully so that she does not overtire the client. Consideration should be given that the person may feel tender in all parts of their body; so be aware of what is best for the client when working so as not to cause too much discomfort. Because of the soreness and pain the client may be feeling, it can also be distressing for the therapist, knowing the client is suffering while trying to cope with such treatments. The therapist can only do her best, giving the client special time and quality of care.

Towards the end of a terminal illness, many clients are very realistic about the outcome. This is where listening skills are essential as well as empathy and understanding. It is during this stage of a person's illness that clients often give even more 'importance' to their 'grooming' than they did in their healthy state. This is possibly due to the deterioration of the body and the need to feel clean and presentable. The deterioration of an ailing body can cause unfamiliar and unpleasant odours which can be stressful for the client. Therefore, helping her to feel good and look good is essential. This is the best support any therapist can give.

Most clients are very knowledgeable about their illness; therefore the therapist will be well informed. One of the most rewarding experiences a therapist will have is the privilege of treating such special people.

In recent years reflexology has become the most favoured therapy among many palliative care clients. Touch and care can offer each client a feeling of relaxation and help to decrease pain and body stress. Whatever therapy a therapist can offer a person in palliative care is very special both to the client and therapist.

CHAPTER 9

The Code of Ethics and the Delicate Balance

CONFIDENTIALITY AND THE CODE OF ETHICS

A 'code of ethics' basically means the moral principles based on rules, regulations and a professional code set out by a governing body related to the practitioner's modality and which must be followed. Members must abide by the rules and work within the specialised field in which they are qualified. Any practitioner failing to follow these rules, or acting unprofessionally, may find their membership terminated and possibly have difficulty practising, due to a record of misconduct.

Some issues that may be displayed on a 'Code of Ethics' chart are as follows:

1. Confidentiality.

2. Working within the boundaries of her qualified field.

3. Updated skills and professional standards of work.

4. No condemnation among colleagues or another member of the profession.

5. No condemnation of another practitioner in front of a client.

6. No discussion of a client's treatment to another client or patient.

7. No involvement with a client's personal problems.

8. No involvement in a personal relationship with a client.

9. Professionalism in conduct at all times.

10. Strict observance of hygiene practice and safety regulations at all times.

Other rules may be added to the above list.

It is important for all practitioners to have a full understanding of the code of ethics. Unfortunately this is not always the case, as I have encountered a few health-care practitioners who break the rules, especially confidentiality. Gossip in public about another person is unprofessional. It is most embarrassing to the client who has no choice but to listen to the practitioner discussing another person's problems. This behaviour indicates to the client that the practitioner would similarly discuss her 'affairs' as well. Any practitioner who is in breach of this code is not fit to maintain membership of their organisation or continue practising.

However, there are times when a practitioner needs to discuss a client's condition and this can be carried out by:

- referrals to another practitioner

- discussion of a 'case of concern'

- case studies (client/patient anonymity).

1. *In a referral* (with the clients permission), the practitioner will give the name and relevant details about the client to the referred practitioner. In some cases the referred practitioner may contact the 'referee' practitioner if necessary. This is working within the code of ethics of confidentiality.

2. *Discussion of a 'case of concern'.* This is where a practitioner needs to discuss a client's condition with another practitioner in a case where the practitioner needs some advice. A client's name does not need to be mentioned when discussing a case.

3. *Case studies*. The confidentiality rule is most important and the practitioner must take all precautions that the case studies she is sharing with colleagues do not include the name of the client or any details that may give away the client's identity. It is advisable to obtain the client's permission for case study work, while reassuring her of her anonymity.

Like hygiene practice and safety rules, if the therapist follows the code of ethics in daily practice she should have no problems in maintaining a high standard of professionalism.

THE DELICATE BALANCE

The delicate balance is where the therapist may find herself in a situation trying to decide whether to proceed with treatment to a frail or infirm person. This could be due to many factors:

- The client may have found she can no longer cope with any treatment.

- The client may not be aware of what is being done to her.

- The client's illness has worsened.

- The client may have developed a high sensitivity to touch.

- The client does not wish to have any further treatment.

When a client chooses not to have treatment, do not try to persuade her to have it. This can be difficult for the therapist, especially when a relative is adamant for the client to have treatment. In this case, the therapist must decide what is best for the client, not what is best for the relative.

> Often I had to 'let go' of a client because I knew she was not enjoying the therapy, and sometimes was in a lot of pain. Another reason was that the client could not cope with the treatment her family members wanted her to have. Some family members were disappointed that I did not continue with the

client's therapy, but ultimately I gave preference to the client's wishes. I knew I had made the right decision.

However, there are times when the therapist may find she has a client who is not very responsive and wonder whether or not to proceed. This can happen more frequently with clients who suffer with dementia. There are a few things the therapist can do to ascertain whether the client wants to continue with treatment. Examples:

- Greet the client by her name. (Sometimes the client may open her eyes and say 'hello', or simply open her eyes; this may be a signal for the therapist to continue.)

- If the client has responded, tell her who you are: identify yourself.

- Ask if she wishes to have her treatment (she may either agree or become more confused).

If the client has responded to the above questions, then the therapist may proceed. If the client has not, set up the equipment on a table with which the client may be familiar, and have it close so she can see what is happening. Proceed again with the above steps and see what response the client offers. The nursing staff may be able to tell the therapist this is normal behaviour for the client and that she will probably enjoy having some pampering. This is where the therapist will have to decide whether or not to go ahead. The therapist must feel confident that she has made the right choice.

> This situation could be 'tricky', as I have been caught out a few times with 'quiet' clients. I remember one day I approached a client who was lying in her bed waiting for me to give her her regular manicure. On this day, I could not get any response. She appeared to be asleep and I thought it would probably be better to leave her and come back another time. As I started packing my bag to leave, the client held up her hand, looked at her fingernails and then looked at me. I asked her again, did she

want her nails done. She just nodded her head and closed her eyes, leaving her hand held up above her head in readiness for her manicure. Learning the signals from frail clients comes with experience. When you have been treating clients, especially those with dementia, for a period of 18 years you get to know many signals from non-communicative clients.

Other incidents the therapist may face with regular clients who have dementia are that they become confused, wondering who you are or thinking you could be someone else. If a client is confused, be clear who you are and what treatment you are going to give. Sometimes it can take a few minutes for the client to understand what is going to happen. I have found it best to have nearby something recognisable for the client, such as my cosmetic bag or some cosmetic accessory.

I had a few clients on my list who could not remember me but were happy to come along to the salon in the nursing home to have whatever was offered to them. When they entered the salon and saw the cosmetics on the table I had laid out before them, they soon remembered that I was going to give them their facial and manicure and were pleased to have their treatment.

Most dementia clients I have treated enjoyed having their beauty treatments and many always looked forward to their next appointment, even though they could not always remember who I was.

OVER-SERVICING

Older frail clients do not always require weekly appointments with beauty therapy or, in some cases, with natural therapies. This is because some therapy treatments may be too much for them to cope with if they are given too frequently. I have found fortnightly appointments are satisfactory for most. Leaving time between appointments can give extra time for healing, should the client have ongoing skin problems and fingernail disorders. For example, if the fingernails have been cut too short or coloured nail polish has stained the nails, or there has been an infection, healing time will give the fingernails or the skin problems a chance to recover. The other reason is that cosmetic application is less invasive, should the client be sensitive to the cosmetics. Finance can also be a reason. Some older clients are on a limited budget and could not afford to have regular weekly treatments. However, many have managed to afford three-weekly to monthly appointments.

> It is more likely for relatives who are financially well off to pay for a client's regular treatments.

A client assessment and information from the RN will give the therapist a better idea of how often the client will be able to have treatments. The RN will be able to notify the therapist if a client is suitable for therapy or not; this includes non-communicative clients.

CONCLUSION

The most valuable lesson I have learned over the years while treating frail people is that the more I know, the more I realise how much I do not know. I have found that this is a challenge in itself. In researching topics on illness, medication and cosmetic applications, I have been assisted by clients who have allowed me access to their own individual experiences in clinical trials. This has increased my confidence in treating frail persons in care. I am grateful for those who have been with me along this journey, inviting me into their lives and reliving their happy memories, passing on their knowledge and ideas, all of which as helped me to grow. The experience I have gained has provided me with a very 'worthwhile' and rewarding career. There will be times that a therapist may feel she is too challenged and possibly may feel 'out of place'. Allow the clients to guide you in helping them, they know what is best. Always listen to what they are saying and 'observe'.

I trust that this book will be of value to many therapists by encouraging them to take this journey, enabling them to introduce new methods and ideas upon which they can improve. Careful personal grooming and relaxing therapies will help to restore a sense of dignity and pride into the lives of the 'forgotten ones', the people in care.

REFERENCES

Better Health Channel (2013a) *Arthritis*. Available at www.betterhealth.vic.gov.au/bhcv2/bhcarticles.nsf/pages/ct_arthritis?open, accessed on 26 June 2013.

Better Health Channel (2013b) *Gout*. Available at www.betterhealth.vic.gov.au/bhcv2/bhcarticles.nsf/pages/Gout, accessed on 26 June 2013.

Better Health Channel (2013c) *Multiple Sclerosis Explained*. Available at www.betterhealth.vic.gov.au/bhcv2/bhcarticles.nsf/pages/Multiple_sclerosis_explained, accessed on 26 June 2013.

Better Health Channel (2013d) *Osteoarthritis*. Available at www.betterhealth.vic.gov.au/bhcv2/bhcarticles.nsf/pages/Osteoarthritis, accessed on 26 June 2013.[1]

Bryden, C. (2005) *Dancing with Dementia*. London: Jessica Kingsley Publishers.

Diabetes Australia (2009) *Turning Diabetes Around: What is Diabetes?* Available at www.diabetesaustralia.com.au/en/Understanding-Diabetes/What-is-Diabetes, accessed 26 June 2013.

Ehealth (2009) *What is Pneumonia?* Available at www.ehealthmd.com/library/pneumonia/PNM_whatis.html, accessed on 26 June 2013.

Healthinsite (2008) *Rheumatoid Arthritis*. Available at www.healthinsite.gov.au/topic/rheumatoid-arthritis, accessed on 23 June 2013.

Kulvinskas, V.P. (1975) *Planetary Healers Manual – Survival into the 21st Century*. Connecticut: OMangod Press.

National Institute on Deafness and other Communication Disorders and MedlinePlus (2009) *Hearing Disorders and Deafness*. Available at www.nlm.nih.gov/medlineplus/hearingdisordersanddeafness.html, accessed on 23 June 2013.

Optometrists Association Australia (2009a) *Cataracts*. Available at www.optometrists.asn.au/EyesVision/EyeDiseases/Cataracts/tabid/105/language/en-AU/Default.aspx, accessed on 10 April 2013.

Optometrists Association Australia (2009b) *Glaucoma*. Available at www.optometrists.asn.au/EyesVision/EyeDiseases/Glaucoma/tabid/106/language/en-AU/Default.aspx, accessed on 10 April 2013.

Optometrists Association Australia (2009c) *Pterygium*. Available at www.optometrists.asn.au/EyesVision/EyeDiseases/Pterygium/tabid/108/language/en-AU/Default.aspx, accessed on 10 April 2013.

Optometrists Association Australia (2009d) *Age-Related Macular Degeneration*. Available at www.optometrists.asn.au/EyesVision/EyeDiseases/AgeRelatedMacular Degeneration/tabid/107/language/en-AU/Default.aspx, accessed on 10 April 2013.

Parkinson's Study Group (2009) *Parkinson's disease overview*. Available at www.parkinson-study-group.org, accessed on 22 June 2013.

---

1 This information was provided by the Better Health Channel, a Victorian Government (Australia) website. Material on the Better Health Channel is regularly updated. For the latest version of this information please visit: www.betterhealth.vic.gov.au. For a specific condition, click on 'Conditions and Treatments', scroll down to 'By A–Z of conditions' and click on the first letter of the disease or illness required, for example 'M' for 'Multiple Sclerosis'.

Quit Victoria (2009) *Background Brief: Emphysema and Chronic Bronchitis*. Available at www.quit.org.au.

Reflexology Association of Australia (n.d.) *Home Page*. Available at www.reflexology.org.au, accessed on 10 April 2013.

Southern Cross Herbal School (1997) *Philosophy of Natural Therapies*. Gosford, NSW, Australia: Heteromed Services.

Stroke Foundation (2007) *Effects of a Stroke*. Available at http://strokefoundation.com.au/what-is-a-stroke/effects-of-stroke/, accessed on 26 June 2013.

Tay, S. (2009) *The Carer's Cosmetic Handbook: Simple Health and Beauty Tips for Older Persons*. London: Jessica Kingsley Publishers.

Verity, J. (2009) *What Is Dementia?* Dementia Care Australia. Available at www.dementiacareaustralia.com/index.php?option=com_content&task=view&id=336&Itemid=81, accessed on 10 April 2013.

RESOURCES AND FURTHER READING

ALZHEIMER'S

Alzheimer's Foundation of America
www.alzfdn.org

Alzheimer Society
www.alzheimer.ca

Alzheimer's Society (Dementia Care)
www.alzheimers.org.uk

AROMATHERAPY

Esoteric Oils (2011) 'Aromatherapy for Older People.' Available at www.essentialoils.co.za/elderly.htm, accessed on 7 July 2013.

ARTHRITIS

American Arthritis Society
www.americanarthritis.org

Arthritis Association
www.arthritiscare.org.uk

Arthritis Australia
www.arthritisaustralia.com.au

Arthritis Society
www.arthritis.ca

Tai Chi for Arthritis
www.taichiforarthritis.com

BACTERIAL INFECTIONS

Medline Plus (n.d.) 'Bacterial Infections.' Available at www.nlm.nih.gov/medlineplus/bacterialinfections.html, accessed on 12 April 2013.

BEAUTY THERAPY

Cosmetic Ingredient Review
www.cir-safety.org

Hampton, A. (n.d.) 'Ten Synthetic Cosmetic Ingredients to Avoid.' Available at www.organicconsumers.org/bodycare/toxic_cosmetics.cfm, accessed on 12 April 2013.

BLINDNESS AND DEAFNESS

American Association of the Deaf-Blind
www.aadb.org

Canadian Deafblind Association
www.cdbanational.com

Royal Association for Deaf People
www.royaldeaf.org.uk

CANCER

American Cancer Society Cancer Action Network
www.acscan.org

Canadian Cancer Society
www.cancer.ca/en/region-selector-page

Cancer Council Australia
www.cancer.org.au

Cancer Institute NSW
www.cancerinstitute.org.au

Cancer UK (National Organisations)
www.cancerindex.org

CARERS

Carers Australia
www.carersaustralia.com.au

Carers UK
www.carersuk.org

Young Carers Australia
www.youngcarers.net.au

COLOUR THERAPY

About Colour Therapy
www.altmedicine.about.com
Click on the A–Z under Browse Topic down on the left hand page and select the topic you would like to read about.

Colour Therapy Healing
www.colourtherapyhealing.com

DEMENTIA

Dementia Care Australia
www.dementiacareaustralia.com

DIABETES

American Diabetes Association
www.diabetes.org

Canadian Diabetes Association
www.diabetes.ca

Diabetes Australia
www.diabetesaustralia.com.au

Diabetes UK
www.diabetes.org.uk

FINGERNAIL DISORDERS

Fitzmaurice, M. (n.d.) 'Nail Discolouration and Diseases.' *Ehow Health*. Available at www.ehow.com/about_5127364_nail-discoloration-diseases.html, accessed 12 April 2013.

LUNG DISEASE

American Lung Association
www.lung.org

British Lung Foundation
www.blf.org.uk

Healthinsite
www.healthinsite.gov.au
Click on Health A–Z and select the condition you would like to read about (e.g. Emphysema, Chronic Bronchitis).

Lung Association
www.lung.ca

Lung Foundation Australia
www.lungfoundation.com.au

MASSAGE THERAPY

Australian Association of Massage Therapists
www.aamt.com.au

Massage Today (2013) 'Massage for Older People.' Available at www.massagetoday. com/mpacms/mt/ed_topic.php?id=18, accessed on 7 July 2013.

Mehta, N. and Mehta, K. (2004) *The Face Lift Massage: Rejuvenate Your Skin and Banish Wrinkles*. London: Thorsons.

Widdowson, R. (2003) *Head Massage*. London: Hamlyn.

MISCELLANEOUS

Age Concern
www.ageconcern.org.au

DPS Guide to Aged Care Australia
www.agedcareguide.com.au

Help the Aged
www.helptheaged.ca

Home Instead Senior Care
www.homeinstead.com

Miller, B.F. and Brackman Keane, C. (1987) *Encyclopaedia and Dictionary of Medicine, Nursing and Allied Health*. Philadelphia: WB Saunders Company.

Senior Life Choices
www.yourlifechoices.com.au

Seniors Network
www.seniorsnetwork.co.uk

Totora, G. and Anagnostakeos, P. (1987) *Principles of Anatomy and Physiology*, 5th edition. New York: Harper and Row.

Winter, R. (2010) *A Consumer's Dictionary of Cosmetic Ingredients*, 6th edition. New York: Three River Press.

MULTIPLE SCLEROSIS

MS Australia
www.msaustralia.org.au

Multiple Sclerosis Association of America
www.mymsaa.org

Multiple Sclerosis Society
www.mssociety.org.uk

Multiple Sclerosis Society of Canada
www.mssociety.ca

MUSIC THERAPY

American Music Therapy Association
www.musictherapy.org

Schaeffer, J. (n.d.) 'Music Therapy in Dementia Treatment: Recollection through Sound.' Available at www.agingwellmag.com/news/story1.shtml, accessed 12 April 2013.

NATURAL THERAPIES

Australian Traditional Medicine Society (ATMS)
www.atms.com.au

Natural Therapy Pages
www.naturaltherapypages.com.au

Pure Calma
www.purecalma.com
Articles and information on herbal medicine and other alternative therapies

NUTRITION

Dietitians of Canada (Nutrition for Seniors)
www.dietitians.ca/Your-Health/Nutrition-A-Z/Seniors.aspx

NHS Choices (Eat Well Over 60)
www.nhs.uk/livewell/over60s/pages/nutritionover60.aspx

Nutrition Australia (Nutrition and Older Adults)
www.nutritionaustralia.org/national/resource/nutrition-and-older-adults

OPTOMETRISTS

Optometrists Association Australia (Eyes and Vision)
www.optometrists.asn.au/EyesVision/tabid/77/language/en-AU/Default.aspx

PALLIATIVE CARE

Canadian Hospice Palliative Care Association
www.chpca.net

National Council for Palliative Care
www.ncpc.org.uk

National Hospice and Palliative Care Organization
www.nhpco.org

Palliative Care Australia
www.palliativecare.org.au

PARKINSON'S DISEASE

American Parkinson Disease Association
www.apdaparkinson.org

Parkinson Australia
www.parkinsons.org.au

Parkinson Society Canada
www.parkinson.ca

Parkinson's UK
www.parkinsons.org.uk

REFLEXOLOGY

Association of Reflexologists
www.aor.org.uk

British Reflexology Association
www.britreflex.co.uk

Norman, L. and Cowan, T. (1998) *The Reflexology Handbook: A Complete Guide.* London: Judy Piatkus.

Reflexology Association of America
www.reflexology-usa.org

Reflexology Association of Australia
www.reflexology.org.au

Wright, J. (2003*) Reflexology and Acupressure: Pressure Points for Healing*. London: Hamlyn.

SKIN DISORDERS

Durham, J. (2013) 'Skin Problems for Older People.' *Retirement Expert*. Available at www.retirementexpert.co.uk/SkinProblems.html, accessed 12 April 2013.

SPECIAL AIDS

ActiveLite Mobility Systems
www.activelite.com/mobility_aids.htm

Mobility Aids Australia
www.electricscooter.com.au

Mobility Store (Mobility Aids)
www.mobilitystore.co.uk

STROKE AND HEART DISEASE

American Heart Association
www.heart.org/HEARTORG

British Heart Foundation
www.bhf.org.uk

Heart and Stroke Foundation
www.heartandstroke.ca

Stroke Association
www.stroke.org.uk

Stroke Foundation
www.strokefoundation.com.au Tai Chi

UNWANTED FACIAL HAIR

Pearce, C. (n.d.) 'Causes of Facial Hair in Older Women.' Available at www.ehow.com/facts_5002326_causes-facial-hair-older-women.html, accessed on 12 April 2013.

VIRAL INFECTIONS

Derm Net NZ (2002) 'Viral Skin Infections.' Available at www.dermnetnz.org/viral, accessed on 12 April 2013.

Gawkrodger, D. (2000) *Dermatology*, 3rd edition. Edinburgh: Churchill Livingstone.

Viral Infections (n.d.) 'Viral Infections.' Available at www.viralinfections.org, accessed on 12 April 2013.

INDEX